Case Management Review and Resource Manual:
The Essence of Case Management
2nd Edition

Kathleen Moreo, RN, Cm, BSN, BHSA, CCM, CDMS, CEAC
and Anne Llewellyn, RN,C, BHSA, CCM, CRRN, CEAC

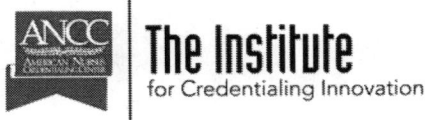

ANCC
AMERICAN NURSES CREDENTIALING CENTER

The Institute
for Credentialing Innovation

Dedicated to every case manager who seeks to improve his or her practice

ISBN 10: 0-9768213-1-1
    13: 978-0-9768213-1-1

Case Management Review and Resource Manual: The Essence of Case Management was completed by Professional Resources in Management Education, Inc. (PRIME)

First Printing—April 2001
2nd Edition—March 2005

Please direct your comments and/or queries about the content to:
k.moreo@primeinc.org or call (954) 718-6055

The health care delivery system is a volatile marketplace demanding superior knowledge, clinical skills, and competencies from all case managers. Autonomy of practice as well as career marketability and mobility in the new century hinge on affirming the competencies and outcomes of health team members. The knowledge base of case and care management is expanding, and while care has been taken to ensure the accuracy and timeliness of the information presented in the *Case Management Review and Resource Manual: The Essence of Case Management*, you are advised to always verify the most current national treatment guidelines and recommendations, and to practice in accordance with professional standards of care with regard to the unique circumstances that apply in the many practice situations. In addition, every effort has been made to insure accuracy including changes to government regulations and developments in product information provided by pharmaceutical manufacturers. However, it is the responsibility of each case manager to practice in accordance with professional standards of care.

Therefore, the authors, editors, American Nurses Association (ANA), American Nurses Publishing (ANP), American Nurses Credentialing Center (ANCC) and the Institute for Credentialing Innovation cannot accept responsibility for errors or omissions, or for any consequences or liability, injury and/or damages to persons or property from application of the information in this manual and make no warranty, express or implied, with respect to the contents of the *Case Management Review and Resource Manual: The Essence of Case Management*.

Published by:
The Institute for Credentialing Innovation
American Nurses Credentialing Center
8515 Georgia Ave., Suite 400
Silver Spring, MD 20910-3492
Phone (301) 628-5000 FAX (301)628-5342
Internet Address: www.nursecredentialing.org
e-mail: revmanuals@ana.org

Introduction to the Continuing Education (CE) Contact Hour Application Process for *Case Management Review and Resource Manual: The Essence of Case Management, 2ⁿᵈ Edition*

The Institute for Credentialing Innovation now offers the continuing education contact hours for this manual online at www.Nursingworld.org, the American Nurses Association's Web site. This process involves answering approximately 50 questions that test knowledge of the information contained within this manual. The continuing education contact hours can be completed at any time and a certificate can be printed from the Web site immediately upon successful completion of the test.

The *Case Management Review and Resource Manual: The Essence of Case Management* is designed to meet the following objectives:

1. Describe the concepts, process, goals, principles and model of case management as practiced in various healthcare settings.
2. Analyze five areas of practice where, with an understanding of data management, the case manager can advance the quality of care, improve access to care and achieve cost savings.
3. Explain six of the major reimbursement systems, their key differences in delivery of healthcare services and their interface with the practice of case management.

Upon completion of this manual <u>and</u> the online CE test, a nurse can receive a total of 25 (twenty-five) continuing education contact hours. **The entire process—online test and evaluation form—must be completed by December 31, 2008 in order to receive credit.**

To begin the process, please e-mail revmanuals@ana.org *or* go to the ANCC website at www.nursecredentialing.org for specific instructions.

Your patience with this new process is greatly appreciated.

Inquiries or Comments

If you have any questions about the CE contact hours, please e-mail The Institute at: revmanuals@ana.org. You mail also mail any comments to Barbara Burnham, RN, BSN, MA, Editor/Project Manager, at the address listed below.

Duplicate CE Certificates

Once you have successfully passed the CE test on NursingWorld, you may go back and re-print your certificate as often as you wish.

The Institute for Credentialing Innovation
American Nurses Credentialing Center
Attn: Editor/Project Manager
8515 Georgia Avenue, Suite 400
Silver Spring, MD   20910-3492
Fax: (301) 628-5342

The American Nurses Association is accredited as a provider of continuing nursing education by the American Nurses Credentialing Center's Commission on Accreditation and approved by the California Board of Registered Nursing, Provider Number CEP6178.

MEET THE AUTHORS

Kathleen Moreo, RN, BSN, BHSA, Cm, CCM, CDMS, CEAC is co-founder and President of Professional Resources In Management Education, Inc since 1994. She has 25 years' experience as an independent case manager, and is an accomplished international speaker and author in case management, managed care, rehabilitation, and health care business management. Ms. Moreo earned her BSN and a Bachelor of Professional Studies in Health Care Administration from Barry University, Miami, Florida. She holds both nationally recognized case management certifications: Cm from the American Nurses Credentialing Center and CCM from the Commission for Case Manager Certification. She also holds national certifications as a disability management specialist (CMDS) and as an environmental access specialist (CEAC). Ms. Moreo is a national past president of the Case Management Society of America (CMSA) and inaugural chair of the Case Management Society International. In 2001, she was honored by CMSA as Distinguished Case Manager of the Year. In 2002-2003, Ms. Moreo co-authored the update to the CMSA Standards of Practice for Case Managers and served as co-chair of the CMSA Standards of Practice Update Task Force. She currently is a member of Sigma Theta Tau International Honor Society of Nursing; an active committee member of the Academy of Managed Care Pharmacists (AMCP); and a member of CMSA.

Anne Llewellyn, RN,C, BHSA, CCM, CRRN, CEAC is co-founder and Vice President of Professional Resources In Management Education, Inc since 1994. She has 20 years' experience as an independent case manager, and has worked as a critical care nurse in Pennsylvania and Florida. Ms. Llewellyn earned her Associates Degree in Nursing from Hahnehmann University, Philadelphia, PA and her Bachelor of Professional Studies in Health Care Administration from Barry University, Miami, Florida. She holds national case management certification (CCM), as well as national certification as a certified rehabilitation registered nurse (CRRN), and is nationally certified as an environmental access specialist (CEAC). Ms. Llewellyn is a past president of the Case Management Society of America (CMSA) as well as being a member in the American Nurses Association and the Emergency Nurse Association.

TABLE OF CONTENTS

Chapter 6 Utilization Management   87

Chapter 7 Disease Management   97

Chapter 8 Health Care Legislation   107

Chapter 9 Reimbursement Systems   115

Chapter 10 Legal and Ethical Issues   129

PREFACE

Historically, case management has been the nemesis of a convoluted health care system. It is the catalyst of patient-centered care, serving as a critical communication link and an advocate amidst high tech care delivery. It is the source of best practices and the scrutiny of payers, where it is viewed both as a necessary process for compliance and a calculated method to lower risk. It is seen as a parody by some physicians, and as an ally to others. It is the darling and the devil of legislators. It is continuously explored, engaged, and re-engineered worldwide as a solution to global health care problems involving cost, quality and access of health care.

A search of the literature reveals several books and manuals on the topic of case management. Yet, practicing case managers and emerging practitioners argue that few guides sufficiently address the consistent process of case management despite practice setting, pay system, professional affiliation, or patients served. **This review book is intended to fill that void.** It is intended to embrace the essence of case management across the continuum of care. It is a window to explore the common theme of varying case management definitions, and to illustrate the true case management process amidst challenges, complexities, and changes in our dynamic health care system.

Case management is not rocket science. It is not a mystery to be solved by astute consultants or ambitious government legislators. Human nature sometimes causes us to over-complicate the process and practice of case management because it is difficult for us to accept an effective solution to a global health care problem.

Effective case management promotes access to care, containment of escalating costs, enhancement of quality products and services, identification or creation of viable alternative care plans, and patient awareness regarding self-determination and empowerment. Case management epitomizes best practice in the continued quest for a health care system based on wellness rather than illness.

In fact, case management's positive effect nationwide and even worldwide is so far-reaching that analysts continuously seek to dissect the process and the practice. What they find is a variety of emerging and maturing case management and care coordination systems that are all somewhat effective but highly complex and variable. Most systems include levels of utilization management, disease management, resource management, and discharge planning within the umbrella of case management and care coordination services. Many are struggling with reporting of and evaluation of measurable outcomes. Few have identified a system that can remain fixed within our changing health care climate.

Despite the fluidity of case management, fundamental principles remain inherent to the practice. The most effective, consistent process of case management is one that promotes quality, cost-effective care at the most appropriate time, in the least restrictive environment. Methods to achieve this process in all practice settings will be presented throughout this book.

Case management is dynamic. Its strength lies in its fluidity. Seasoned, advanced case managers often "break the rules" of conformity to effect positive, cost-effective change for their patients which, in a rippling effect, can enhance the entire health care system. Good case managers are comfortable in their role as change agents.

This book is an effort to review the true process of case management, and in doing so, to send out ripples of best practice to every corner of the health care delivery system. It is an effort to take the mystery out of case management. It is a framework for how to use streamlined, core functions of case management across the care continuum to optimize patients' and communities' wellness. It intends to put you into your case management role with the comfort to be a change agent—to transport you to a higher dimension in your case management process and practice.

We hope you enjoy the ride!

Kathleen Moreo, RN, Cm, BSN, BHSA, CCM, CDMS, CEAC
Anne Llewellyn, RN,C, BHSA, CCM, CRRN, CEAC

CASE MANAGEMENT CONCEPTS AND PROCESS

1

The process of case management has emerged as a recognized intervention to control spiraling health care costs as well as to ensure quality healthcare to those who are most at risk. The practice dates back to the early 1900s when the coordination of services for the sick and poor as well as the conservation of public funds was a recognized need. Case management is rooted in a long history of social work and nursing efforts.

An example of how the social work model brings to light the case management process can be gleaned from a demonstration project that was known as Chicago's Hull House. Chicago's Hull House was founded in 1889 to offer a variety of programs for the immigrant populations. The major contribution that came from this program, and remains significant to the practice of case management today, is the recognition of the worth of individualized treatment, and the need to assist patients toward self-support and self-sufficiency. The program established that for effective outcomes to be achieved there is a need for a trained staff as well as the systematic collection of data.[1]

The nursing case management model traces its roots to Lillian Wald, a leader in public health nursing, who worked in New York City in the early 1900s. Wald's accomplishments set the principles on which today's case managers have been able to build. Specifically, Wald showed the importance of early identification of those who are at risk for developing complications from illnesses and injuries, the need for proactive education for the patient and their families, and the importance of viewing the patient and the family holistically in order to improve quality of life and contain health care costs.

Wald's efforts were demonstrated in the Henry Street Settlement House established in 1893. Wald organized the Settlement House to care for the elderly, pregnant, and disabled of New York City's lower East Side. Wald and her nurses visited those in need in their homes to educate about germs, transmission of disease, and the importance of good personal hygiene. They provided preventive, acute, and long-term health care to all with whom they worked. The programs were so successful that they expanded to include assistance with housing, employment, and education for exceptional and mentally challenged children.

Other efforts led by Wald, which remain a major focus for case managers specializing in the occupational health setting, were those to improve the health of employees in the workplace. Wald challenged major industries to provide health inspections of the workplace to protect workers from injuries. She was able to persuade corporation executives that protecting the health of their employees made good business sense. She encouraged them to implement preventive medicine and to have nursing or medical professionals at the work site at all times.[2] Wald's philosophy remains a cornerstone to the current practice of occupational health case management.

Today, as case managers continue the efforts of former leaders, the need to control escalating costs and manage epidemiology is still important. However, the practice of case management has changed as public policy has changed. Case management has also kept pace with advances in technology that have extended life beyond expectations. The practice of case management is viewed from both disciplinary and interdisciplinary viewpoints and is incorporated in various settings throughout the continuum of care. Individual disciplines have adopted and practiced case management, generally deriving definitions based on discipline-specific models.[3] It is important to remember that no one discipline "owns" the practice of case management. This concept has caused controversy within the industry and has led to five different but similar nationally accepted definitions. As the practice of case management matures, the goal should be that there is one definition to unite the practice. Until that time, case managers must be cognizant of their own discipline's definition, model, and practice setting. The following section will list the approved national definitions from the major organizations that support the practice of case management.

DEFINITIONS

The approved definition of nursing case management by the American Nurses Association (ANA) and adopted by the American Nurses Credentialing Center (ANCC) states:

"Nursing Case Management is a dynamic and systematic collaborative approach to providing and coordinating health care services to a defined population. It is a participative process to identify and facilitate options and services for meeting individuals' health needs, while decreasing fragmentation and duplication of care, and enhancing quality, cost-effective clinical outcomes. The framework for nursing case management includes five components: assessment, planning, implementation, evaluation, and interaction."[4]

The Case Management Society of America (CMSA) supports a multi disciplinary role of case management, rather than focusing on case management as a function of nursing or social work. The definition of case management updated in 2002 and published in the CMSA *Standards of Practice for Case Management 2002* is:

"Case management is a collaborative process of assessment, planning, facilitation and advocacy for options and services to meet an individual's health needs through communication and available resources to promote quality cost-effective outcomes."[5]

The approved definition of social work case management by the National Association of Social Work (NASW) states:

"Social work case management is a method of providing services whereby a professional social worker assesses the needs of a client and the client's family, when appropriate. The case manager arranges, coordinates, monitors, evaluates and advocates for a package of multiple services to meet the specific client's complex needs. A professional social worker is the primary provider of social work case management. Distinct from other forms of case management, social work case management addresses the individual client's biopsychosocial status, as well as the state of the social work system in which case management operates. Social work case management is both micro and macro in nature: intervention occurs at both the client and the system levels. It requires the social worker to develop and maintain a therapeutic relationship with the client, which may include linking the client with systems that provide him or her with needed services, resources and opportunities. Services provided under the rubric of social work case management practice may be located in a single agency or may be spread across numerous agencies or organizations.[6]

The approved definition of nursing case management by the American Board of Occupational Health Nurses (ABOHN) states:

"Occupational health case management is the process of coordinating the individual employee health care services to achieve optimal quality care in a cost-effective manner. The case manager establishes a provider network, recommends treatment plans that assure quality and efficacy while controlling cost, monitoring outcomes, and maintaining a strong communication link among all parties."[7]

The approved case management definition by the Association of Rehabilitation Nurses (ARN), and adopted by the Certified Rehabilitation Registered Nurse credentialing body (CRRN) states:

"Case management is the process of planning, organizing, coordinating, and monitoring the services and resources needed to respond to a client's health care needs".[8]

Organizations representing other health care disciplines are also in various stages of evaluating the role of case managers in specialized settings. The American Association of Respiratory Care (AARC), for example, provides an information package for therapists interested in becoming case managers. Although there are multiple definitions that define the process of case management, the common thread that connects each discipline is the goal of case management; that, regardless of setting, each case manager advocates for those at risk and strives to provide quality, cost-effective care at the appropriate time in the least restrictive environment. The philosophy of case management is that all individuals are eligible for case management services regardless of the ability to pay for that service.

It is important to remember that not everyone requires case management. Applying an accepted business principle, such as the Pareto principle, to health care, it is estimated that 80 percent of the health care resources are spent on 20 percent of the population.[9] This ratio reflects the population that would benefit most from case management services. For case management to be successful, early identification of people who are at risk, and then stratifying them according to need, are essential. Identifying of those at risk is a process that is a way to ensure that those at risk do not fall through the cracks of a fragmented and complicated health care system. Risk stratification will be discussed in more detail in Chapter seven.

Case management services are implemented to meet the needs of the individual. Gaining permission and establishing trust with the patient and the family are also important, since case management is a voluntary service. The cooperation of the patient and the family ensures better compliance with the treatment plan, which is necessary to achieve successful outcomes. The following terms describe the essential functions of the case management process.

Assessment

Assessment is the first essential function of the case management process. Assessment is an organized, multidimensional process by which the case manager, through interaction with the client, significant others, and health care providers, collects and analyzes in-depth information about the dimensions of physical, psychological, socio-cultural, spiritual, cognitive, functional, and developmental abilities, economic issues, and lifestyle.

To perform this task, the case manager collects information from relevant sources that the case manager feels might be important to uncovering the needs of the client. Examples of sources that may provide a holistic picture of the patient include: the family, other health care institutions, professional caregivers, employers, public health records, and school and military records. The case manager should obtain a written release of information from the patient/family to gather this material to ensure patient confidentiality. More information on this topic will be addressed in Chapter ten.

An in-depth evaluation of the information provides valuable insight regarding the current and past history of those who are at risk or who may benefit from case management services. This process also allows the case manager to see how effectively the health care system has been used in the past. In many cases, over- or underutilization of service can be discovered. Many times, clients use the health care system in inappropriate ways and do not benefit from services that do not meet the true needs of the patient.

The chronic pain patient is an excellent example of over-utilization of emergency and acute care services in an attempt to seek help. Despite using a great deal of resources, outcomes are often not successful since the true aspects of pain have not been addressed. By having a holistic view, the case manager can identify those patients who are currently suffering from chronic pain, or those who may be at risk for developing chronic pain, and work to promote access to specialists who can accurately diagnose and apply interventions that begin to meet those needs. The information that the case manager collects during the assessment process is evaluated objectively and critically to identify needs, clarify and determine realistic goals, and seek potential alternatives to the current plan of care.

A complete and comprehensive assessment is critical to facilitate a successful case management plan. Strategies for successful data collection include the review of existing records, interviewing the patient and/or family, and observing the interaction between the patient and the family and community. Keen assessment skills are needed to enable case managers to make an accurate assessment of the patient's status, particularly if the assessment is done telephonically.

In an attempt to gather pertinent information in an organized manner, many settings have instituted detailed tools to aid in the initial assessment. These tools provide a guide to focus on the specifics of the patient's status, current problems, and medical history, and provide a view of the patient's perception of his/her current health status. Assessment screening tools can aid the case manager to obtain a clearer understanding of the needs of the patient and the opportunity to incorporate educational programs. These tools can also identify the readiness of the patient to learn, and assist with implementing practices that would improve adherence to the plan leading to an improvement in the patient's overall health status. A detailed description of screening tools will be presented in Chapter four.

Planning

The second essential function to the case management process is planning. Planning is the process by which the case manager develops a patient-centered, evidence-based, interdisciplinary plan of care based on complete analysis of data.[10] The case manager collaborates with the health care team and the patient to develop an individualized plan of care. The plan should be action-oriented and time-specific. The goal of the plan is to provide quality care that enhances outcomes and reduces the payer's liability. A comprehensive plan prioritizes the needs of the patient to meet the immediate needs and moves the patient through the continuum of care.

Depending on the timelines of the case management plan, it may be started in one setting and continued into another setting. The ideal scenario is that the same case manager follows the patient from one setting into another setting. However, oftentimes each level of care results in a new case manager. For example, a patient transitioning from an acute care setting into a rehabilitation facility, and then back to home with the support of home health care could have at least four case managers coordinating his/her care—the acute care case manager; the rehabilitation case manager; the home health case manager; and the payer case manager. It is important that the case manager responsible for transferring the patient from one setting to another ensures that detailed information is provided regarding what has been done, what the future plan is, and why the transfer is taking place. Documentation presenting the rationale for the transfer is important to ensure continuity of care between providers.

A key question that the case manager should ask and be able to answer is, "What is the clinical evidence that allows this patient to move safely from one setting to the other?" The answer to this question provides the rationale for the transfer. There are specific rules that apply to the transfer of patients from one setting to another, so it is important for all case managers to be aware of the policies and follow them to guard against inappropriate transfers. Information on health care legislation involving transfers will be covered in Chapter eight.

The case manager works with the treatment team in developing the plan and obtains approval for the plan of care from the treating physician, the patient and the family, and the payer. Depending on the payer source, the case manager may need to gain authorization for the plan. This is especially true in the area of workers' compensation, as well as with some commercial managed care organizations. Authorization is needed prior to the implementation of the plan and needs to be considered in the planning phase. It is important that the case manager be aware of the cost of the plan that is being constructed to ensure that the plan is cost effective in meeting the needs of the patient. If funding is not available, and the services are needed, the case manager will work through the chain of command to gain approval or negotiate in order to manage the financial aspects of care.

The case manager must recognize that denial of payment for services from the payer is not the final word. As an advocate for the patient, the case manager must look at what is medically necessary and strive to find resources to safely ensure that those services are met. This may mean asking for an exception to the benefit plan, utilizing community resources, or extending the patient's stay in the current setting. A safe and appropriate discharge is essential to any case management plan. This process falls under the umbrella of resource management, which will be covered in more detail in Chapter five.

The case management plan is written, keeping in mind the goals that are to be achieved as a result of specific treatments or services provided. Setting goals gives the plan structure and a way for the case manager to report outcomes in an organized manner. Goals should be appropriate to the individual patient, measurable, attainable, relevant, and time orientated. The individual as well as the family should be part of the development of the immediate short- and long-term goals. By working closely with the family, the case manager is able to assist them in gaining an understanding of the diagnosis and treatment plan as well as the need to understand the relationship between lifestyle, personal habits, attitudes, and well-being. An outcome that a case manager can claim from this collaboration is adherence to the plan of care. Adherence is pivotal to achieving care that is high in quality, reduces health care costs, and attains desired heath outcomes. The effectiveness of the case management process is based upon the linkages between interventions, adherence, and outcomes.[11]

Implementation

Implementation is the third essential function in the case management process. Implementation is the execution of the specific case management activities and interventions that lead to accomplishing the goals set forth in the plan. Implementation includes pro-active activities that include: intervening, delegating, facilitating, and communicating with all involved. Once the plan is developed and approved by the treating physician, the payer, and the patient and family, the case manager implements the plan of care. Using negotiation skills, the case manager works to ensure that services begin in a coordinated manner among the various providers, the patient, and family. Through careful planning, knowledge of resources, and appropriate communication, duplication of services is avoided and fragmentation is reduced. The result of this effort is that the patient receives care that is appropriate, timely, and cost-effective.

The ability of the case manager to implement a successful plan of care will be influenced by his/her level of education, training and clinical expertise. For example, a masters' prepared case manager has specialized skills and knowledge that include, but are not limited to, the ability to effect change; perform critical analysis; promote patient/family autonomy; build positive relationships; and understand/interpret research for enhanced decision making. They can utilize these skills sets when implementing challenging plans of care to maximize successful outcomes.

Coordination and Interaction

The fourth essential function of the case management process is coordination/interaction. The process of coordination and interaction is essential and inherent to all phases of the case management process. These components consist of organizing, securing, integrating, and modifying the resources necessary to accomplish the goals set forth in the case management plan. As part of this process, the case manager must be aware of the cost of the current care as well as the cost of the care that has been recommended, to ensure that interventions recommended are cost-effective. When possible, community resources should be used. The case manager must also be cognizant of, and compliant with, regulations, standards, and legislation at the local, state, and national levels. Competency skills that are essential for the case manager to be effective in coordinating an individualized plan of care are effective communication skills, collaboration, assertiveness, and cooperation with all parties.

As mentioned earlier, coordinating a safe and effective plan of care is critical to the success of the plan. The case manager must verify that the individual and the family understand the plan of care, and that the various providers who have been contracted understand their roles in the process. The case manager validates that interventions are consistent with the established plan of care, and that the plan is implemented in a safe and timely manner. The case manager who initiates the plan, if not following the case through the continuum of care, should make a follow-up call to be certain that all aspects of the plan are in place. By proactively addressing problems regarding the plan, the case manager can intervene early to make changes as needed. If problems are found, the case manager assesses the situation and develops measures to address the situation.

In many cases, once the patient leaves a specific setting, such as the hospital, interaction with the case manager ends. In other cases, a new case manager may take over the case. The important point to remember is that a smooth transition is possible when communication and collaboration occurs among all parties The patient and the family should be given instructions about how to follow up if they have questions or concerns about any aspect of the plan of care. Documentation of all case management activities is the final detail in this process.

Monitoring and Evaluation

The final essential elements in the case management process are monitoring and evaluating. To ensure that the plan of care is meeting the goals set, the case manager monitors the plan of care on a continuing basis by gathering information from the providers involved to show that the plan implemented is effectively meeting goals. Proactive monitoring of the plan ensures that the patient is making progress toward the desired outcomes. If progress is not being made, modifications or changes to the plan in its entirety, or in specific components, are made as needed.

Evaluation provides the case manager an opportunity to improve the plan of care in a proactive manner. The evaluation process is part of continuous quality improvement standards that organizations and accreditation bodies require. In addition, the evaluation process gives the case manager time to review providers to see that all services for which contracted are provided in a manner consistent with the organization's standards. The evaluation process is measured by achievement of the specific goals that meet the patient's needs in a timely and cost-effective manner.

GOALS AND OBJECTIVES OF CASE MANAGEMENT

The primary goal of the case management process is to provide services that ensure appropriate, quality care for individuals who are at risk, in a timely and cost-effective manner. Case management services are individualized, holistic, and meant to enhance self-care through the continuum of care. The objectives that the case management process strive to achieve include:

- assist the client and family to achieve optimum function;
- coordinate the delivery of care, decrease fragmentation and assure appropriate use of resources;
- enhance the quality of life for the individual patient/family;
- improve and facilitate interdisciplinary communication and planning;
- help to strengthen the family unit when injury and illness strike;
- maximize the health of consumers by increasing health care education that promotes wellness;
- proactively identify problems and needs, and implement services that provide appropriate high-quality care to meet the individualized needs of the patient/family.[12]

PRINCIPLES AND RELATIONSHIPS

Case management is a dynamic and fluid process that spans the continuum of care. Those who enter the practice bring with them specific skills from their individual disciplines that, when taken collectively, enhance the practice overall. To achieve successful outcomes, each case manager must strive to acquire skills and knowledge to improve practice, and to build relationships with the diverse group of people with whom the case manager will interact. To make these skills viable, a brief description of terms that pertain to the practice of case management is provided. These terms will also be covered in greater detail throughout this manual.

Accountability

As professionals, case managers are held responsible or accountable for the implementation of the case management process within their scope of practice. Thus, it is important that case managers practice within the scope of practice of their respective disciplines. In addition to the individual scope of practice, professionals who engage in case management have standards of practice that document criteria that guide the practice. In 1995, The Case Management Society of America (CMSA) promulgated standards of practice to provide guidance for excellence in case management. A committee of experts in the field re-visited the standards in 2001 to determine their ongoing application to the dynamic practice of case management. The CMSA standards are used today by many entities in the U.S. and abroad to ensure and measure case management accountability within the variety of settings where case management is practiced. Information regarding legal issues of accountability pertinent to the practice of case management will be covered in Chapter ten.

Advocacy

The definition of an advocate, according to the American Heritage Dictionary, is one who pleads or defends the cause of another.[13] Advocacy is the common denominator that unites case managers, regardless of practice setting or professional discipline. As advocates, case managers individualize each plan of care to meet the specific needs of clients and families. An important aspect of the case management process is the manner in which the case manager supports and educates the patient and the family. The end result of this effort is to empower the patient to be self-reliant and to self-advocate. Advocacy will be discussed later in this chapter and in Chapter ten.

Autonomy

Autonomy is an ethical principle defined in the CMSA Ethical Statement as, "A form of personal liberty or action when the individual determines his or her own course of action in accordance with a plan of care chosen by him or herself."[14] The principle of autonomy also involves the recognition that the patient has a right to make an informed decision about his or her own health care decisions. For this to occur, patients are entitled to honest, accurate information about all aspects of their care. Case managers must adhere to the wishes of patients and not impart their own judgments. Addressing and resolving ethical issues pertinent to autonomy will be covered in more detail in Chapter ten.

Collaboration

Collaboration is an essential skill that the case manager needs to unite the members of the health care team, and others who are integral to designing a plan of care for an individual patient. Collaboration by the case manager fosters consistency, which reduces fragmentation and duplication of services. Effective collaboration ensures patient and provider satisfaction, an important outcome that all health care professionals strive to achieve. The timely delivery and sensitive handling of information by the case manager are essential to ensuring patient confidentiality and relevant decision-making. When pertinent information is communicated to providers in a timely manner, the case manager ensures that decisions are made with full information, thus decreasing duplication of services.

Cost Effectiveness

Case managers attempt to coordinate cost-effective, quality care as the basis of the case management process. By accurately assessing and developing an effective and efficient plan of care, and monitoring the plan proactively, the case manager initiates steps to decrease over- and underutilization of services that cause waste and fragmentation, and which contribute to rising health care costs. Documentation of cost-effective care is important for all case mangers to report as part of the case management process.

Continuity of Care

Continuity of care is viewed as an uninterrupted or unbroken course in the care of a patient. To provide continuity of care for a patient, especially for the patient with chronic illness or injury, case managers must use professionals who can provide medical care and services that meet the patient's specific needs in an organized and timely manner. Communication between providers is essential for continuity to be maintained. Equally important is that the patient and the family be informed about all aspects of care, so that continuity can be maintained. The case manager can act as the point of contact, to ensure that communication is enhanced and a seamless plan is achieved.

Critical Thinking and Problem Solving

As case managers increase their presence in the health care system, the need for critical thinking and the ability to problem-solve becomes more crucial. To achieve effective outcomes in today's health care environment, the case manager must have skills that ensure problem identification in a proactive manner, and timely resolution. An organized approach uses strategies to ensure effective problem solving. These strategies include;

- Identify the issue;
- Understand each party's issue;
- List possible solutions;
- Evaluate the outcomes;
- Select an option or options;
- Agree on contingencies, monitoring, and evaluation.[15]

The traits needed by case managers to critically think and problem-solve include excellent communication skills, organizational skills, flexibility, and creativity. By using critical thinking skills, the case manager is able to identify problems, investigate solutions, and work to ensure that a timely resolution occurs to maintain continuity of care.

An example that illustrates this point is when a managed care case manager, who is working with a young child and his parents, has learned that the child will need a bone marrow transplant due to acute lymphacytic leukemia. The case manager, in speaking with the treating physician, discovers that the best place for the transplant is a center of excellence in another city. Once the transplant is done, the child will need to stay in the area for at least three weeks to be nearby in case complications occur. The case manager knows that this information is going to cause a hardship for the family, since they have other children and have no real support system.

In speaking with the parents, the case manager suggests that the mother accompany the child, and that the father apply for leave from work under the Family Medical Leave Act (FMLA). This way, he will be able to take time off to be available for the other children without jeopardizing his job. The case manager investigates information on the FMLA. She knows that the father works for a large company and will be eligible for this benefit. The case manager explains information about the FMLA to both parents and assures them that their situation is an example of why the Act was passed. The father agrees to file for a leave of absence under FMLA to remain at home with the other children. Having solved this critical issue, the case manager calls the facility where the transplant will be done to see what information they need to begin the transfer process.

Interpersonal Communication

Verbal and written communication skills are essential. As professionals at the center of the team, case managers must have the ability to interpret complex, detailed clinical and financial information, and disseminate that information to individuals who need to know—both verbally and in written form. The case manager must be able to take a vast amount of information and summarize it, without distortion or insinuating personal judgment. When talking to professionals, the case manager must have concise questions that allow professionals to understand what is being asked, and to provide information to specific questions.

Case managers need to be sensitive to the time of other professionals. There is a popular expression that case managers should keep in mind: *Your emergency is not my emergency.* Case managers must respect the time of others when asking for information that will help them. Case managers also talk with a variety of people, ranging from highly educated professionals to average laypersons. It is important, when communicating, to consider the educational level of the other person. When communicating with people from different cultures, translation services may be needed to ensure that the person you are talking with understands the information being communicated. Another communication skill, essential for the case manager to have, is the ability to listen. The case manager will learn a great deal of information by listening and observing those with whom they interact. More information on communication skills is covered in Chapter two.

Information is also obtained and transmitted in written form. Many times, the case manager may compose letters that will be mailed, faxed, or sent by e-mail to the treating physician or provider, asking for information to help clarify or update the plan of care, or offering details of a revised treatment plan. It is important that case managers be aware of legislation concerning patient privacy that applies to all forms of communication, and to comply appropriately. Further information on the patient privacy and security act will be covered in Chapters eight and ten.

Accurate documentation is an essential form of communication to describe outcomes and improve the process of case management. Written documentation is viewed as the permanent record that specifies, summarizes, analyzes, and synthesizes verbal and nonverbal data that support the work and time that a case manager gives to each patient. Data management will be covered in more detail in Chapter four.

Negotiation and Conflict Resolution

Effective case managers are skillful negotiators. The basic skill for successful negotiation is the ability to build solid relationships. The level of trust between parties, knowledge of the parties, and the flexibility of those involved in the negotiation process influence the success of any negotiation. When case managers take the time to understand what motivates each person who is part of the process, negotiations are more likely to be successful. The effective case manager takes time to examine and understand the impact of the case management plan on all those involved.

Managed care has decreased the need for price negotiations due to provider contracts that are set up in advance. Today, the case manager is viewed as the negotiator of care rather than the negotiator of costs. This view has broadened the focus to allow the case manager to look at the entire process, rather than only at the narrow focus on costs. As part of the broad focus, the case manager still has the obligation to ensure that the services and products put into place are medically necessary, priced appropriately, and delivered with high quality service. In the case of a patient who needs multiple medications after a heart transplant, the case manager should negotiate prices with three vendors within the network to ensure that the patient is receiving the most cost-effective price, since the patient will need to be on these medications for life. If the nurse case manager is able to negotiate a lower rate, the savings negotiated are reported as an outcome. More information on this topic will be covered later in this chapter.

Negotiation skills allow the case manager to resolve conflicts that may arise. As health care professionals, case managers are required to interact with people during very intimate and stressful times.

Astute case managers have the opportunity, using their diverse interpersonal relationship skills, to recognize a potential conflict and to put measures in place that address and resolve conflicts in a manner agreeable to all. To resolve conflicts, the case manager must be able to encourage and maintain open communication and facilitate a positive flow of ideas among all parties with whom interactions occur.

To put conflict resolution into focus, step into the shoes of a workers' compensation case manager who faces a common situation that involves returning an injured worker to work. In accomplishing this goal, the case manager must interact with the employer, the employee, and the treating physician. An experience that is common, once the treating physician decides that an injured worker is able to return to work but requires accommodations, is to convince both the employer and the employee that return to work is possible. The case manager may encounter an employer who states that return to work cannot be accommodated because of restrictions that the doctor has specified as necessary. In this case, the worker is reluctant to return to work, since he has worked only as a mason. He states he is willing to try, but wants to be certain that he won't suffer another injury.

In speaking with the employer, the case manager finds that the reason that the employer is resistant to having the employee back is that he was not much of a "go-getter". "What can I give him to do, that won't waste his time or mine?" is a common question that the case manager hears. To resolve this conflict, the case manager explains to the employer the benefits that he will derive from bringing the employee back to work. To prevent a potential conflict, the case manager reviews with the employer the restrictions that the doctor has given the injured worker, and asks if there is any type of work that the employee can perform in the office. The employer remembers he has a drawer filled with addresses of potential clients that he has not had time to contact. He formulates a plan to bring the injured worker into the office, and have the worker make preliminary calls on which he can then follow-up, if interest is expressed. The case manager takes this opportunity to explain that, by bringing this employee back to work, the company's future workers' compensation rates may not increase. Also, morale will be improved when other workers see that the employer is willing to accommodate an employee who was injured. Finally, the injured worker, who is being paid whether he works or not, will be more productive to the employer by being at work, rather than sitting at home watching TV. The case manager also notes that the injured worker has not yet retained an attorney. Showing support to the injured worker, the employer may prevent any legal action from occurring.

The result of this conversation was that a date was set for the employee to begin the office job. The case manager advises the employer to put the offer to return to work in a letter to the employee regarding the start date, and the work that he will be doing. The case manager assures the employer that he/she will stay involved to assist with any problems that may arise. The case manager informs the employee of this, who is pleased about the opportunity to work in a different position, and believes that he can do a good job. The case manager documents this information, showing that the patient can return to work now that the employer is able to accommodate him safely in the work setting. The savings reported regarding an early return to work show the cost savings associated with reduction in lost time. Information regarding return to work and modified jobs will be covered in more detail in Chapter three.

Outcomes-Focused Care

Once an individualized plan of care is crafted, the case manager is responsible for initiating the interventions and monitoring the plan's effectiveness. Specifying expected outcomes at the onset of care planning allows the case manager to evaluate the effectiveness of those outcomes. From a global view, to integrate outcomes into the quality improvement process, all information about outcomes should be reported, whether they are successful or not. Identifying all outcomes allows providers and practitioners to focus on systems structure, and to make changes as needed to improve both systems and individualized practice. Outcomes are discussed in greater detail in Chapter four.

Performance Improvement

Performance improvement is a process that allows health care organizations to determine how their services are meeting the needs and expectations of those who use services. By critically evaluating clinical, financial, and utilization data, information is obtained that allows performance measurements to be implemented throughout the continuum of care. The goal of a performance improvement program is to ensure that the systems in place are able to meet the patient's needs and expectations. This is achieved by measuring outcomes such as patient satisfaction, improvement in functional status, and increase in quality of life indicators.

Service Integration

Service integration is a method used by integrated delivery systems to provide and arrange for coordinated services to a designated population. An efficiently integrated delivery health system has three principal components: financing, management, and delivery. The relationship among these components is critical to everyone involved in the practice of health care. Integration allows practitioners to meet the needs of the public regarding access to services, efficient management of resources, and the delivery of services in a timely manner. Access to the delivery of health care services needs to be designed so that services can be easily accessed anywhere along the continuum of care. The case manager plays an integral part in this process by ensuring that services and products are coordinated and used appropriately to meet the needs of the consumer in a cost-effective manner.

Timeliness

For case management to be successful, early identification of those who are at risk is essential. In cases of sudden catastrophic illness or injury, early referral to case management services is essential to ensure that the patient is admitted to the appropriate facility that will meet his/her medical needs. For those who suffer from chronic illness or progressive disease, the need for case management services is determined by how the patient and the family are handling their specific challenges. Screening tools such as SF-36 provide the health care team with information about the patient's perception of the illness. This information allows those who need assistance in improving their health status to be identified early, thus avoiding or minimizing potentially costly problems.

Timeliness is also important for patients who are not currently registered in the health care system, such as patients who use only the hospital emergency department (ED) as their primary care centers. The emergency department case manager, by a review of data, can identify patients who use the system on a routine basis, and begin to assess the individual needs of patients. An example is the diabetic patient who is seen in the ED several times for problems related to dizziness and blurred vision. In this case, the case manager would be able to talk to the patient about these problems, review lab results, and discuss the clinical picture with both the ED physician and the patient, to gain a better understanding of how the patient is managing the illness. The case manager may learn that the patient has problems with access to a primary care physician, financial challenges, and/or lack of education about diabetes. Timely identification and referral to appropriate resources will result in decreased fragmentation of care, improved quality of care, and reduced costs associated with misuse of resources.

ROLES

The role that the case manager performs varies, depending on the setting but, in general, all roles strive to promote collaboration with clients by assessing, facilitating, planning, and advocating to improve the quality of health care each person receives. To be familiar with various roles, the following terms are defined.

Advocate

Advocacy is the thread that unites all those who practice case management. As an advocate, the case manager supports the patient in meeting goals and ensures that those involved in caring for the patient understand the patient's individualized needs. The case manager advocates for the patient to ensure that all members of the health care team work collaboratively to incorporate services/products for the patient throughout the continuum of care. The patient's best interests are represented when the case manager advocates for such issues as ensuring access to needed services, investigating funding resources, and identifying treatment alternatives that are safe, less restrictive, and coordinated in a timely manner. More information on the case manager's role as an advocate is discussed in Chapter ten.

Consultant

The case manager serves as a consultant to members of the health care team who may need assistance with patients, or with issues that arise during the course of treatment. The case manager can assist with hard-to-find resources and solutions to problems that providers wish to explore for those patients who may not necessarily need a case manager on an ongoing basis. The case manager also consults with other health care professionals, such as vocational counselors, when negotiating to return a patient to work. In some cases, special testing or intensive evaluation may be needed to find out what type of gainful employment may be right for an injured or disabled person. The vocational specialist is trained to perform these services. To obtain such services, the case manager speaks with the treating physician to obtain an order for the consultation, and then seeks authorization from the claims adjustor to implement this service. The case manager also collaborates with employers and school officials when facilitating return-to-work or school for an injured worker or a child who has sustained an injury or illness. The case manager can make recommendations for accommodations that are appropriate for the person to safely reintegrate into the community. Issues relating to consultation will be covered in more detail in Chapters two and five.

Educator

An important role that the case manager performs is that of educator. The case manager educates on many levels and for various reasons to ensure that the process is efficient. The case manager educates the health care team so that they understand how the process of case management works in today's health care system, as well as what resources are available through the continuum of care. The case manager educates the patient and the family on an ongoing basis about issues pertaining to symptom management, disease progression and prognosis, and injury/illness prevention. The case manager can translate confusing medical terms and procedures, and assist in bringing logic to a confusing system. The case manager, who has a keen understanding of the diagnosis, clinical goals, and community resources, assists the patient and family to understand the diagnosis and treatment plan. This allows the patient to make informed decisions regarding the course of care. More information on informed decisions will be discussed in Chapter 10. Buy-in by the patient and the family maximizes the ability of the patient to comply with the plan, which can eventually result in positive outcomes. Finally, case managers have an obligation to self-educate to maintain and improve their clinical and case management competencies.

Liaison

The case manager as a liaison unites the health care team, the payer, and the community with the patient and family. Balancing the needs of all requires qualities such as the ability to build positive relationships, assertiveness, empathy, organizational skills, and the ability to effect change. An example of this role can be illustrated by understanding the important role that the social worker plays in the health care system.

The social worker is part of the health care team who acts as a liaison between patients/families and the various professionals and agencies who can provide resources. Many times, patients have a need for community support because of pressures of illness or injury. The social worker has expertise in resource management, enabling them to mobilize and maximize resources so that the family is directed and connected with needed services.

An example that occurs often in long-term care is the ability of the social worker to coordinate services for an older patient who is being discharged to home after rehabilitation from a fractured hip. The patient is able to live independently, but needs some assistance with shopping and cleaning her home. Elderly services are found in the community to meet this need, allowing the woman to be discharged safely, in a timely manner.

Facilitator

As a facilitator, the case manager implements a plan of care and ensures that the process moves forward. The case manager also works to identify and remove barriers to the plan of care. Issues that may arise are proactively addressed to prevent delays in care. In the case of system problems, the case manager identifies these from trends that become apparent based on variance tracking. The case manager is usually the one who is best able to track trends throughout the entire system. The case manager brings the problem to the attention of the appropriate person or committee, reports the issues, and facilitates changes to address and correct the problem. This is an integral part of the continuous quality improvement plan that most organizations have in place. More information will be presented on variance tracking in Chapter four.

Mentor

The case manager assumes the role of mentor as a way to expand the practice. An experienced case manager can mentor new professionals entering the field. At times, employers hire professionals who have little or no case management experience. An experienced case management professional should assist the new case manager with an introduction to the company or institutional philosophy, policies and outcomes pertinent to the practice of case management. The experienced case manager can assist the new case manager during the orientation period in understanding the case management process in general terms, as well as how it relates to the individual practice. Entrepreneurial case managers may work with organizations that wish to implement or improve case management programs in provider organizations. In this case, as a mentor or consultant, the case manager goes into a setting, assesses the strengths and weaknesses, and makes relevant recommendations to improve the overall care management process.

Researcher

The last role to be covered in this section is the role the case manager plays in research. The masters' prepared or doctoral level case manager can participate in and contribute to the field of research as an advance practice professional. Research is the means of enhancing the body of knowledge to elevate the practice of case management to a recognized profession. As the practice of case management evolves and matures, it is important for those who have expertise in the area of research to use research methodologies to refine and validate the practice. However all case managers should utilize research findings which build a strong evidence-based approach to their practice.

Case management roles can be very different depending upon the health care setting. Some examples of different case management roles, defined by setting, are provided in the following examples.

Brokered Case Manager

The brokered case management model fosters the procurement of needed resources and services for the client.[16] The brokered case manager, or independent case manager, contracts directly with a managed care organization, or the patient/family, to ensure that the patient receives the necessary treatment and services. The brokered case manager in this model serves as the liaison between the patient, the provider(s), and the payer. The brokered case manager carries out all case management functions and provides direct services, coordination, and advocacy by linking patients to appropriate settings, providers, and services. The brokered case manager develops a comprehensive plan of care, and negotiates barriers that may prevent patients from accessing needed services. The primary goal is to increase the ability of patients to receive the right services in proper sequence and in a timely manner.

A brokered case manager may be used when the payer is not getting information about a specific patient who has suffered a catastrophic injury or illness. This allows the payer to better understand the plan of care and prognosis for the patient. The managed care organization (MCO) will contract with a brokered case manager to make an on-site visit to see the patient, speak to the family, review the medical record, and discuss the plan of care and prognosis with the treating physician. The brokered case manager will then work collaboratively with the acute care case manager and the payer case manager, to appropriately meet the needs of the patient.

A brokered case manager is viewed as the "eyes and ears" of the MCO in this example. An early referral to a brokered case manager in catastrophic cases ensures that the patient is proactively managed, and that the provider and the payer address needs in a timely manner. Brokered case managers can also be hired directly by the patient/family to assist in coordination of services. Because case managers are independent practitioners, they should maintain their own malpractice insurance, since they are not covered by a specific employer, and act as independent contractors. Information about malpractice insurance will be provided in Chapter ten.

Provider Case Manager

The provider case manager is a professional who works for a specific provider to assure proper utilization of services in a quality manner that is cost-effective for the payer and provider. The role of the provider case manager increased in demand when the risk shifted from the payer to the individual provider. More information will be presented about the shifting of risk and its effect on health care in Chapter nine. The goal of the provider case manager is to assure that the services requested meet the needs of the individual patient and are used in a cost-effective manner. Patient and family education is a priority for the provider case manager so that the patient/and or family may learn to self-manage. The provider case manager is found in all settings along the continuum of care.

Payer Case Manager

The goal of the case manager who works in the payer setting is to manage appropriate access to services and promote the use of cost-effective alternatives. In some instances, the case manager in the payer setting may restrict access to high-cost services and treatments to control utilization, and thereby reduce costs. To avoid delays, case managers and providers who collaborate with payers should provide appropriate documentation for all products, services, and treatments. This information supports the validity of the request and allows the payer case manager to review the information and match criteria against standards they use to make utilization decisions. If they are unable to justify the request, payer case managers can take the information through the chain of command. This may be done if the cost or services are outside the patient's benefit plan, but are warranted. A cost-benefit analysis that "spells out" the benefit, as well as the cost of services, products, and treatment will be helpful for the case manager to have in advocating for alternatives. More information regarding cost benefit analysis will be discussed in Chapter four.

Outcomes for the payer-based case manager depend on the availability of appropriate, cost-effective alternatives, and the case manager's ability to control the cost to the payer. The case manager who works in this setting often faces ethical issues due to the demand to provide quality care, yet the need to control spending. Case managers must use their clinical and critical thinking skills when following policies that are set regarding how care is delivered and paid. The chain of command should be folso that the case manager is not the final word in a controversial decision. Each payer has an appeal process that should be used to communicate clearly what is being denied and why. Information on the appeal process will be covered in the section covering utilization management in Chapter six.

Self-Care Case Manager

The self-care case manager is the patient or the family. The family may act as the case manager for those patients who, because of age, mental or physical disability, or other deficit, are unable to advocate for themselves. The goal for all professional case managers is to educate and empower the patient and the family toward self-care, to enable them to become their own case managers.

These examples demonstrate that the health care setting will greatly influence the role a case manager assumes. Models and settings for case management are further discussed in the next section.

MODELS AND SETTINGS

Today, case management is found in every setting of the health care system. The current settings within the continuum of care represent the various resources available to health care professionals to meet patients' needs. Depending on the setting, different models of case management may exist. The challenge case managers encounter is how and when to use the available resources in an appropriate and timely manner.

Unfortunately, there is a misperception in this country that to receive the best care possible hospitalization is needed. This concept has slowly changed in recent years, with advances in technology and systems management that make it possible for many treatments and procedures to be performed in other venues. As a result, patients who come to the hospital have higher acuities, and patients who are discharged are more complex. The following section is an overview of the various settings that exist in the current health care system, and a description of the functions performed by the case managers who work in these settings.

Acute Care

Acute care hospitals in the U.S. represent the largest segment of health care settings. Hospitals and related physician expenditures traditionally account for the majority of health care spending. In 1998, thirty-three cents of every dollar was spent just on hospital care.[16] Because of the rising costs of health care spending, a radical redesign has been imposed on all aspects of the health care system, with the acute care setting being hardest hit. The government, payers and accrediting organizations have imposed many rules and regulations that have caused hospital administrators and chief financial officers to continue to struggle for ways to comply, yet remain profitable.

Today, it is not easy to "get admitted" to a hospital. For a patient to be admitted, the treating physician must ensure that the patient meets specific criteria that support the need for admission. Managed care settings, as well as other payer systems, require that utilization procedures be implemented in acute care settings to ensure that patients admitted meet specific criteria, and that those confined to the hospital continue to meet the criteria for acute care. The purpose of the acute care setting is to diagnose and treat those who are too sick to have procedures and treatments performed in alternative settings. Documentation which includes medical necessity for testing and procedures is needed from the team following the patient in the hospital. This information is submitted to payers to evaluate whether the care given meets the required criteria.

The case manager who works in acute care must ensure that the procedures planned are performed in a timely manner, and results obtained, interpreted, and addressed promptly to allow the health care team to determine the future plan of care. The duties that case managers perform differ from setting to setting, according to the size and philosophy of the health care institution. Many acute care settings have sophisticated case management programs that address all aspects of the delivery of care, while other settings are less complex and may focus only on specific functions, such as discharge planning or utilization review.

Despite the type of program that exists, the emphasis on appropriate utilization of services and cost containment continues as a high precedent in all acute care hospitals. Many payer organizations send external case managers into the acute care setting to control or direct resources. Health care providers across the continuum of care are responding by developing policies and procedures to protect patient confidentiality, while improving systems that allow them to comply with payers. Acute care case managers are charged with proactively identifying patients who will not meet specific criteria or who have social/financial problems that cause them to have extended or frequent stays. Once obstacles are identified, the case manager can begin to address the needs of the patient and/or family by implementing an individualized plan of care.

Those professionals who practice as acute care case managers usually are nurses and social workers. Institutions often use the combined skills of both professions to effectively meet the needs of the population served. Acute care settings obtain various accreditations to show the community and the payer(s) that they meet standards set by organizations such as the Joint Commission on Accreditation of Healthcare Organizations (JCAHO). These accrediting organizations in turn look to case management departments to show that care is coordinated through each delivery segment of the acute care setting.

Episodic Care

In many cases health care is practiced and received in an episodic manner. A case manager in an episodic setting is usually limited regarding the amount and types of interventions that can occur. This is primarily because the patient will only be seen in the facility or organization for a limited period of time directly related to the episode requiring care. For example, a case manager in the hospital will provide episodic interventions for an elderly patient with a hip fracture during the five days the patient is receiving care. As plans are being made to discharge the patient, the case manager may transition the patient's need for ongoing case management interventions to the payer case manager or the home care case manager. Although the hospital based case manager may follow-up with the patient after discharge, his/her primary interventions are completed by the acute care case manager at the time the patient was discharged.

Episodic care often results from an accident or an event that occurs due to complications or setbacks from a chronic condition, such as exacerbation of chronic obstructive pulmonary disease or congestive heart failure. In these cases, the acute care case manager may be able to work with the patient or family to identify triggers that cause setbacks, and educate the patient and family as to ways to avoid exacerbations. If the acute care setting has an integrated delivery system, then the case manager may be able to make a referral to a community-based case manager, who can follow the patient after discharge. Many times this is effective in decreasing episodic events and enhancing quality of care.

Post-Acute Care

As the term implies, post-acute care occurs after an episode of care in the acute care setting. It is the responsibility of each acute care case manager or health care professional to document the rationale regarding why someone is moving from one setting to another setting. The case manager or discharge planner is responsible to ensure that the transfer is performed in a safe and efficient manner. It is important that the patient is medically stable for transfer and agrees to the plan of care. A physician must be willing to follow the patient in the new setting, and a report is given to the receiving facility concerning the current status of the patient. Once this information is obtained, and appropriate papers signed, a copy of the entire medical record should accompany the patient so that the receiving facility has information on what occurred in the acute care setting. The case manager or the discharge nurse should be available for any questions that arise as a result of the transfer.

An example of a how the post-acute care setting is used is shown in the case of a 72-year-old widow who fell at home and sustained a fractured pelvis. The patient was seen in the ED and admitted to the hospital for stabilization. After four days, the orthopedic physician recommended discharge. The case manager found, when talking to the patient, that she lived alone and had no support system. The case manager discussed this with the treating physician, who agreed that the patient could be transferred to a sub-acute facility for rehabilitation, to ensure safety and to increase function. Arrangements were made for a physiatrist to accept the patient and a bed was made available for the patient. The patient was informed of, and agreed to, the transfer. The case manager began the process of copying the record and setting up transportation. The patient was transferred to the facility, where she was able to receive physical therapy, gain strength and function, and restore self-confidence that was lost due to the fall. After three weeks, the patient was able to ambulate using a walker and was ready for discharge from the sub-acute facility.

Sub-Acute Setting

As demonstrated, many times a patient does not need the intensity of an acute care setting and can receive care in a less intensive setting. Some MCOs have systems set up that allow for direct admission to a sub-acute facility from the home or an emergency department if the patient has needs that do not meet criteria for acute care but also not stable enough to go home.

An example of this is an 80-year-old man who is admitted to the ED with shortness of breath, sweating, and bilateral pedal edema. The ER physician orders oxygen, a diuretic, and a foley catheter as well as lab work, an ECG, arterial blood gasses, and a chest x-ray. After a few hours, the physician evaluates the patient. He is sitting up, eating a light lunch, and talking with the patient in the next bed. His labs, ABGs, and ECG are within normal limits, but because of the presence of some fluid in the lung, and the patient's past history of heart disease, the ED physician recommends admission. The MCO calls the Hospitalist to evaluate the patient, and it is decided that the patient is stable for transfer to a sub-acute facility for observation. The patient is agreeable to this, so arrangements are made for the transfer.

Sub-acute facilities are also used by many managed care settings for those patients who may require rehabilitation, but do not currently meet the requirements for acute rehabilitation at the time a transfer is deemed medically necessary. An example of this scenario is a 68-year-old diabetic patient who has had a stroke and requires rehabilitation. Because of her overall condition, the patient is not physically able to endure three hours of acute rehabilitation, so arrangements are made for the patient to be transferred to a sub-acute setting to allow her to regain some strength in a less intensive setting. The sub-acute setting may be used as a "bridge" that enables the patient to gain sufficient physical strength to be able to meet the three-hour rehabilitation requirements of the rehabilitation center.

Rehabilitation

Rehabilitation is another setting where many patients receive care after an injury or an illness that affects their ability to care for themselves, including complications or deficits that affect activities of daily living (ADLs). Patients who suffer from a CVA, spinal cord injury, traumatic brain injury, amputation, or other illnesses or injuries can benefit from a stay in a rehabilitation setting. Rehabilitation facilities have specialized staff who can address the physical, functional, and psychological areas affected by a catastrophic injury or illness. Many rehabilitation facilities elect to meet strict criteria set by the Commission on Accreditation of Rehabilitation Facilities (CARF), which ensures that the facility has the staff and the expertise to meet the services provided.

Rehabilitation can be performed in an inpatient setting, a transitional setting, or in the outpatient setting. Each setting has specific criteria, and the rehab team, led by a physiatrist, will usually make the determination as to when the patient is ready to move from one setting to another. The case manager who works in the rehabilitation setting is considered a specialist in rehabilitation case management.

Skilled Nursing

Skilled nursing facilities are specialty centers that care for patients who have long-term needs and are unable to care for themselves. Many of the patients who reside in these centers are elderly, but skilled nursing facilities can also focus on the child who has severe disabilities. The goal of these centers is to maintain the maximum health status for the residents, and care for them in a humane and compassionate manner. On the whole, most skilled nursing facilities strive to deliver good care for residents. In the cases of those which do not, many are under scrutiny by the government and the public to improve services to their residents. Family members must be encouraged to visit those in skilled care facilities, since many times patients cannot advocate for themselves. If abuse is suspected, information should be reported to the state agency that oversees skilled care facilities in the state where the facility is located. Case managers who work in skilled care facilities should ensure that current advance directives are in place, so that, if a patient must be transferred to an acute care setting, this information can be communicated. More information on reporting of abuse and on advance directives, is discussed later in this section and in Chapter ten.

Community-Based Care

In 1999, the national expenditure for health care topped $1.2 trillion dollars.[17] In order to contain spending in view of our aging population, the American health care system is undergoing a change from a focus on illness to one that focuses on wellness. With this shift and the need to contain costs, there is also a shift of care from the acute care setting to community and home settings. This trend places tremendous pressure on the health care professional to educate consumers about how to change behavior, and to encourage consumers to assume more responsibility for their care when they have an illness or an injury. The following are some of the services available to meet the needs of the patient and family when care moves into the community.

Home Health Care

Patients are now being sent home with complicated medical problems. Case managers and discharge planners must be cautious when discharging a patient to home, to ensure that the family is prepared to safely handle the needs of the patient. To assist with this challenge, many payers are working with home care agencies in their networks to evaluate patients and families so that when discharge is determined, the patient/family are ready. The desired outcome that can be achieved is that the patient is able to receive needed care at home in a safe and cost-effective manner.

The needs of the home health patient will determine the level of care required. The case manager coordinating discharge to home for a ventilator-dependent patient works with an experienced high-tech home care agency to facilitate care for both patient and family. A specialized home care agency should have professionals with expertise and appropriate credentials to provide both the high-tech nursing and the high-tech respiratory care to meet the patient's needs. In the same vein, an elderly man being discharged home who is having changes in mental status due to progressive Alzheimer's disease, will require a lower level of intensity to meet safety needs. The key to understanding the needs of the patient and family is to ensure that a comprehensive assessment using an interdisciplinary team identifies all needs required to transition the patient from the inpatient setting to the home setting.

Proactive, collaborative discharge planning will assist in determining the needs of the patient, and in finding the correct setting for the patient, once medically stable. Partnering with home care organizations to meet various needs of patients helps the case manager or discharge planner to ensure that the plan of care is safe. Teaching is a key component when preparing the patient and family for the return home, and helping the family to understand and to perform the care needed. In long-term cases, it is particularly important that attention is paid to the caregiver, since this role is difficult and often overlooked. The home care case manager must advocate with the payer and, many times, with members of the patient's family, to ensure that respite care is incorporated into the treatment plan to prevent burnout of the caregiver.

Durable Medical Equipment

Durable medical equipment (DME) companies are organizations that supply equipment and other supplies that a patient will need when care is provided in the home. Many DME companies provide what is called a "one-stop-shop." Through these companies, the case manager can order supplies, medications, coordinate nursing care, and arrange transportation to take the patient to and from the doctor's office. Some DME companies supply only medication and nursing care, while others simply specialize in equipment and supplies. The type of company the case manager uses will depend largely on the payer source and the specific needs of the patient/family. The case manager or discharge planner should verify whether the patient has insurance or how services/products are going to be financed, prior to coordinating services. If the patient or family cannot afford equipment, community resources can be investigated.

It is important that the patient and/or family understand how to use any equipment or supplies that are delivered to the home. Education can be provided directly from the DME provider, or by a specialist/consultant. An example would be a patient who is discharged with end stage cardiomyopathy. A technician who has been trained by the company to use the equipment may set up oxygen for the patient, and instruct the patient regarding potential hazards of oxygen use in the home. In another case, a respiratory technician may be required to provide respiratory therapy and give detailed instructions for ongoing therapy to the family/caregivers of patients who suffer from chronic respiratory conditions such as cystic fibrosis and asthma. More information on this subject is covered in Chapter five.

Hospice

Hospice is used to assist the patient and the family when a chronic condition or an injury is likely to result in death in the "near" future, and the patient does not want aggressive treatment that will prolong life. Today, every patient who enters a health care setting is asked about advance directives. Advance directives give people a way to communicate in advance about how they want to be treated when end-of-life is imminent. Advance directives must be recognized and respected by the health care team. Education of consumers as to how advance directives are used is also important to prevent unnecessary and unwanted procedures, according to the patient's wishes. Patients are encouraged to bring a copy of their advance directives with them each time they are admitted to a facility. They should also supply a copy of the advance directives to the primary care physician. More information on advance directives is covered in Chapter 10.

Case managers are required to inquire about the wishes of those who are terminally or chronically ill, and ensure that those wishes are respected. Consulting with hospice care professionals is one way the case manager can assist the patient and the family to address end-of-life issues. The current focus of hospice has shifted from looking at the patient who is assessed as terminally ill, to working earlier with patients who have progressive chronic illness, such as COPD or cancer, to address issues concerning the end of life. Hospice then assists both the patient and the family in proactive planning for impending death.

Long-Term Care

The focus of long-term care is on specific populations that require professional or personal services on a recurring or continuous basis due to aging, or the presence of a chronic or permanent physical or mental impairment. Populations that fall under this category include the elderly, because of their age and inability to function; adults who suffer from chronic illness or catastrophic injuries that have left them dependent; and children who require long term care because of devastating injuries, illnesses, or congenital defects.

Professionals who work with older people to address their long-term care needs are known as geriatric care managers. The geriatric care manager is called upon many times by the individual client, the family, or trust officers to assist with coordination of medical care, transportation, and personal issues such as paying bills, shopping, housecleaning, and general upkeep of the home for those who can no longer perform these tasks. The geriatric case manager coordinates these services for the individual to ensure that the individual is safe and receiving appropriate services that provide maximum independence. Payment for services provided by the geriatric case manager are usually made on a fee-for-service basis to whoever contracts the service. Adult children of aging parents often contract directly with geriatric care managers. Many companies that specialize in long-term care insurance are now employing geriatric care managers to assist with care, once a policy is activated. Today, many people are planning ahead and purchasing long-term care policies that will be available to them if and when the need arises. Information on this type of policy will be discussed in more detail in Chapter nine.

Children with chronic conditions also have special health care needs and require frequent use of medical services, equipment, supplies, medications and access to community resources. Children who fall into this category are children with birth and genetic anomalies, complications from birth that have left them disabled and dependent, and various accidents that have caused permanent damage, such as near-drowning, and brain and spinal cord injuries. Case managers who work with this population either in private practice or through a government agency such as Medicaid or Children's Medical Services, are most successful when relationships are formed among families, physicians, and nurse care coordinators, since the needs of children are so diverse. More information on aspects of chronic illness will be covered in Chapter seven.

Patients who are over 21 years of age and under the age of 65 with long-term needs often are covered by private health care insurance. The payer-based case manager usually addresses the needs of this population if they have private insurance. Other sources of coverage are found through either Medicaid or Medicare. If the injury or illness resulted from an accident or work related injury, coverage will be provided by a workers' compensation carrier. If the injury was the result of an accident, a legal settlement may have set up a trust that provides money for long-term care needs or medical care not covered by insurance. In such cases, to structure payments, a life-care plan may be needed to outline future needs over a life time, so that funds can be conserved and used efficiently. In cases such as this, a trust officer or bank may be responsible for dispensing funds for long-term care. An independent case manager or the workers' compensation case manager may assist with management of care for this population. If the case manager is not involved, the family or primary caregiver will assume this role. More information regarding life-care plans will be found in Chapter three.

As technology continues to improve and allows people to survive diseases and catastrophic injuries, and our population ages, increased attention is being given to those who require long-term care, to ensure quality and cost containment. As a result of this trend, case managers need to become familiar and comfortable in dealing with the medical, social, and ethical issues that face this population. A proactive approach to assessment, management, and ongoing care and support for those who require long-term care is one way that problems can be recognized early, treatment initiated, and costs controlled. The goal for case managers who work with this population is to strive to ensure that each patient reaches maximum potential, and to educate those with a chronic illness or injury on how to navigate the health care system.

One of the greatest challenges that have come from the growing long-term care population is recognizing and understanding the impact on the caregiver. The National Family Caregivers Association estimates that the value of the services family caregivers provide for "free" is $196 billion per year.[18] Case managers must take time to educate and inform caregivers of creative ways to deal with challenges that arise from caring for the frail elderly, as well as those with catastrophic or chronic conditions.

Assisted Living

Assisted living is a venue that many seniors are moving toward when they can no longer function in their own homes. An assisted living facility allows a person to live in his/her own apartment or room, and then join the community for activities and meals. This type of setting allows the elderly person to remain relatively independent, but allows assistance to be given to ensure safety and proper nutrition.

Many churches or community agencies have set up assisted living programs for those who are catastrophically ill or disabled due to mental or physical conditions. Safety and proactive management to ensure adherence to treatment are important in this population. Assisted living programs can also provide respite care for families who have elderly or disabled persons. These programs allow caregivers to continue to work or have a break from the daily routine while the disabled person is being care for in a safe environment that can stimulate awareness.

Private Duty Nursing

Private duty nursing is implemented in situations when the patient requires one-on-one care. Today, because of the nursing shortage, many families are using private duty nurses to help care for their family members while in the hospital. In this scenario, insurance companies do not typically compensate the cost of private duty nursing, since it is a choice of the family.

Private duty nursing in the home is also effective for children and adults who are catastrophically impaired and require around-the-clock nursing care. A child who has survived a near-drowning and is left in a persistent vegetative state may require 24-hour care to feed, suction, bathe, and provide for all the needs that accompany this type of condition. The family may choose to have the child remain in the home, but needs help to care for the child. Financing this type of care is very expensive and typically not covered under traditional insurance. In the case of legal settlements, structured payments may be set up after a settlement is made to pay for private duty nursing care. Independent case managers can work with the family in need of private duty care, to find an agency that can provide this type of service. The case manager may be able to negotiate a special rate, since the care is ongoing and long-term. Sometimes, nurses are "hired" and work privately to care for a person who requires private duty nursing. In this case, the family is the employer and is responsible to pay the individual nurse, including covering them for such things as workers' compensation and income taxes. The case manager who assists with this type of coordination should encourage the family to seek expert advise about what their responsibility is when undertaking this type of project, to follow the various federal and state requirements that apply to employment.

REFERENCES

1. Conti, R. Nurse case manager roles: Implication for practice and education. *Nursing Administration Quarterly.* 1996: 21,1:67–80.
2. Profiles in Caring. Lillian D. Wald 1867–1940. Available at: www.nahc.org/NAHC/Val/Columns/SC10-4.html
3. Huber, D. The diversity of case management models. *Lippincott's Case Management Journal.* 2000: 25,6:248–255.
4, 10, 11. American Nursing Credentialing Center. *ANCC Board Certification.* Washington, DC. ANCC; 2000:27–28.
5. Case Management Society of America. *CMSA Standards of Practice for Case Management Revised 2002.* Little Rock, AR. CMSA; 2002.
6. National Association of Social Workers. Specialty certification in case management. Baltimore MD. NASW; 1999:1.
7. American Board of Occupational Health Nurses. *American board of occupational health nurse board certification.* Hinsdale, IL; 2000: 2.
8. Edwards, P. *Specialty practice of rehabilitation nurse's core curriculum.* Glenview, IL. Rehabilitation Nursing Foundation of the Association of Rehabilitation Nurses; 1996: 48–49.

9. Vaccaro, P. The 80/20 rule of time management. *Family Practice Management*. 2000: 9,1: 35–38.

12. Mayer, G. Case management as a mindset. *Quality Management in Health Care*. 1996: 5,4:7–16.

13. *The American Heritage Dictionary Second College Edition*. Boston, MA. American Heritage; 1982.

14. Case Management Society of America. *Ethical issues in case management*. Little Rock, AR. CMSA; 1996.

15. Seven steps for effective problem solving in the workplace. Available at: www.conflict-resoultion.net/articles/thicks.cfm

16. Davis, Virginia. Staff development for nurse case management. In: Cohen E, ed. *Nurse Case Management in the 21st Century*. St. Louis, MO. Mosby; 1996;189–201.

17. Ginsberg, E. Medical care in the U.S.—who is paying for it? *Journal of Medical Practice*. 2000: 15,5:34–39.

18. Carson, N. Care for the caregiver. *Take Care! Self Care for Family Caregiver*. 1999: 8,2:1:–12.

CLINICAL PRACTICE

2

Case managers in clinical practice are well positioned to perform the holistic emphasis of care management. They possess clinical proficiency based on their area of study, and are usually comfortable in their specialty domain of care delivery. Their knowledge and the respect of their professional peers are based on experiences obtained in the discipline for which they are professionally licensed or certified. Clinical practice in case management includes the roles of consultant, educator, collaborator, negotiator, researcher, and resource manager.[1] The clinical case manager usually has a caseload for which he/she is directly responsible. Assessment skills, implementation interventions, and evaluations are ongoing. He/she will concentrate on such aspects of a patient's care as functional status; cost of care; mechanisms to measure successful outcomes, such as patient satisfaction; and prevention strategies. The clinical case manager also serves as a resource to clinical nurses and ancillary professionals providing direct care to the patient. He/she will coordinate services with the multidisciplinary team to achieve outcome goals.

A clinical nurse specialist is often utilized in the acute care setting to case manage high-cost, high-chronicity patients who may be identified through the hospital's DRGs. The nurse possesses the skills, knowledge base, and competencies to effectively coordinate care with the multi-disciplinary team to achieve positive outcomes. This individual may also serve as the director of case management, or may direct the clinical performance improvement within the healthcare setting. In another example, a licensed clinical social worker may be utilized as the "problem solver" clinical case manager in a hospital system. On any given day, strengths in behavioral health assessment and resource management may be used to enhance effective discharge planning of a homeless AIDS patient, while experience in crisis intervention assists the emergency room staff to deal with a child abuse case. Meanwhile, the director of nursing on the hospital's medical oncology unit calls on this clinical social work specialist to intervene with grief counseling for the family of a dying cancer patient.

Those clinicians who specialize in holistic bioassessment and functional health planning, such as nurses, usually appear most comfortable learning and assuming clinical case management roles. They are able to perform accurate, ongoing assessments of the patient's disease process to dynamically coordinate necessary changes to the patient's plan of care. They are able to educate the patient/family regarding the disease process, signs and symptoms of complications, and adherence to treatment regimens. They are typically up to date on new treatments and technologies. They also have been educated to emphasize human values, coordinate with the health care team, and act as patient advocate in their role as effective clinicians.

There are a variety of clinicians who have made the successful transition from direct patient care to case management, including occupational therapists, respiratory therapists, social workers, and nurses. Their transition is not made by shirking the knowledge and experience gained as "bedside" clinicians; rather, their professional disciplines serve as the foundation for successful general case management and specialty case management emergence.

Case managers in a specialty or single practice include those who specialize in such disease and injury processes as transplantation, oncology, HIV/AIDS, high risk neonate, pediatrics, chronic pain, traumatic brain injury, and spinal cord injury. Case studies involving these specialty areas can be found at the end of this chapter. Despite specialization, the majority of case managers are generalists, and are in great demand because of their ability to work with a variety of disease processes, comorbidities, age groups, and complex family issues. The majority of clinicians are typically well suited to be generalists because they have valuable work experience in such diverse settings as acute care, intensive care units, emergency rooms, rehabilitation centers, post-acute or home care settings. Clinical practice, therefore, is a significant part of the case management process being used in the current health care system. The most effective clinical case managers are those who continue to keep current with clinical issues once they leave the bedside.

HEALTH PROMOTION AND ILLNESS PREVENTION

The promotion of health and wellness has always been a goal of the clinician. Despite the fact that the health care infrastructure allows for the majority of care to be delivered as a reaction to injury/illness, rather than as a preventive action, society has long believed that all citizens have a fundamental right to wellness. In 1966, national legislation entitled Partnership for Health Act recognized health promotion and illness prevention as a state of complete physical, mental, and social well-being; not merely the absence of disease or injury.[2]

During the years since the tumultuous 1960s, a concept has emerged that health care is more than medical care. Hildegarde Peplau, RN, EdD, Professor Emeritus of Rutgers, the State University of New Jersey in 1974, wrote the following excerpt regarding the evolving theory of health care:

"It is an interdisciplinary enterprise requiring the interdigitation [integration] of knowledge from many sources and the interrelation of many different expert practices of many different independent professions."[3]

Peplau aptly described the case management process, which gathers knowledge and expertise from many sources, and cultivates coordination among interdisciplinary, independent professionals to promote wellness. Another element necessary to promote wellness and prevent illness is the recognition of the physical and psychological characteristics of wellness.

Physical and Psychological Characteristics of Wellness

An example of the differences between physical and psychological wellness includes the orthopedic surgeon who focuses on a geriatric patient's fractured hip. The physician is acutely intent at performing the surgery; monitoring the patient's healing progress in the post-op phase; ordering physical therapy to assist the patient in early and successful ambulation; ordering pain medications and antibiotics to enhance the patient's healing process; planning a safe and early discharge from the acute care setting; and communicating potential signs and symptoms of complications to the patient as a precautionary discharge strategy.

However, the physician often does not consider asking the patient about:

- the home situation, including whether the patient cares for a spouse, lives alone, or even feels safe returning home;
- whether there are elevation changes in the home, or grab bars in the bathroom, or potentially hazardous conditions in the post-op phase, such as throw rugs and poor lighting;
- whether there is someone to assist the patient with activities of daily living during the initial post-hospitalization period, such as cooking and personal grooming;
- whether the patient has a means of transportation to the grocery store, the bank, or doctor's office for the follow-up appointment;
- whether the patient can afford the co-payment on the prescriptions written, or whether the patient even has insurance.

Any of these situations could cause extreme anxiety, fear, and stress for the patient, impairing the patient's psychological wellness. The physician may also not recognize that the patient is demonstrating signs of depression. The depression can either be acute, as a result of post-op challenges, or chronic, stemming from a myriad of potential geriatric challenges unrelated to the surgery.

The case manager is responsible to exercise clinical judgment in determining both the physical and the psychological wellness of the patient. Assessment should be ongoing and should be sensitive to factors that can trigger physical or psychological illness. It is not enough to "cure" the patient physically, or to rely only on one's eyes to assess the patient's health status. Physical health characteristics may be seen with the eye; psychological health characteristics can be sensed with the ear and the heart. This is just one example of when case management is both an art and a science.

HEALTH CARE MANAGEMENT

Assessment tools and diagnostic tests are important components in health care management to assist the case manager and all members of the health care team in determining the patient's physical and psychological functioning. Assessment tools assist the case manager in understanding the patient's disease process, response to the disease, signs and symptoms of complications, perceived health status, and provide an understanding of the patient's behavior in dealing with the complex issues surrounding an illness or injury. More information on assessment tools is covered in Chapter four. Diagnostic tests provide invaluable objective data to assess a patient's physical and psychological functioning.

Physical Functioning

Diagnostic testing is the method of choice by physicians seeking answers to a patient's physical functioning. Diagnostic testing continues to grow in types and numbers, and to become more complex and more readily available in the high-tech world of health care. Currently, health care systems are striving to standardize diagnostic testing based on such pre-determined guidelines as clinical pathways, algorithms and evidence-based practice (see Chapter four). Case managers operating within health delivery systems where standardized guidelines are being used should become familiar and comfortable with the guidelines. Variations in practice will then be more readily identifiable and easier to control.

Case managers cannot be expected to understand the reasoning, mechanics or interpretation for every diagnostic test that is ordered for a patient. However, case managers should have a firm understanding of some of the aspects of diagnostic testing that could directly affect the patient's welfare. A rule of thumb is to consider whether the testing will affect *quality, cost or access issues* for the patient. Questions the case manager can consider include:

- Will hospitalization be required?
- Must testing be performed in a location far from the patient's home?
- Will testing involve time off from work?
- Is testing covered under the patient's insurance plan?
- Are resources available in the community to provide the testing at a reduced rate or free of charge if the patient will otherwise have difficulty assuming financial responsibility?
- Is pre-teaching required to lower the patient's risk at the time of testing, or to optimize the patient's testing and post-test recovery?
- Does the patient have fears, real or imagined, regarding the testing?
- Has the patient been advised of how results will be communicated, and when?

Psychological Functioning

Determining the psychological functioning of a patient involves a different set of diagnostic tools, which case managers are often in contact with as part of the case management care plan. For example, rehabilitation clinicians are very familiar with the Glasgow Coma Scale and the Rancho Scale. These cognitive scales are used in the acute care and rehabilitation settings to determine and to benchmark a patient's level of consciousness and mental function.

Although a generalist case manager may be limited in understanding the complex needs of a head trauma patient, he/she will need to know the patient's level on the Rancho Scale in order to arrange appropriate transfer of the patient to a rehabilitation facility, since most rehabilitation facilities will not accept patients with a Rancho level of less than three. A patient demonstrating a Level three on the Rancho Scale will have localized response, meaning that the patient reacts specifically but inconsistently to stimuli, and may follow simple commands in an inconsistent, delayed manner.

The Rancho Los Amigos Cognitive Scale was developed by the head injury treatment team at the Ranchos Los Amigos rehabilitation facility in California, and was updated in the early 2000's to provide a more comprehensive scale of cognitive function. A total of 10 levels ranks the patient's cognitive function ranging from a Level 1 (no response) to a Level 10 (purposeful and appropriate—modified independent). By contrast, the Glasgow Coma Scale ranks a patient's verbal and motor responses, and eye opening ability. The user adds the assigned numbers to achieve a total score, from a low score of three to a high score of fifteen. The Glasgow Coma Scale is a practical means of monitoring specific changes in a patient's level of consciousness, while the Ranchos Scale measures overall cognitive ability/function and is used widely to gauge ongoing response to rehabilitation treatment/management.

Case managers dealing with a brain injured patient's psychological functioning will also need to understand the purpose and scope of a psychological or neuropsychological assessment. These assessments can gauge deficits experienced by the patient, and as such are key factors in determining whether a patient is an appropriate candidate for transfer to a rehabilitation facility. It is also important for the case manager to understand who is appropriate to perform these assessments, and what members of the health care team would benefit from obtaining a copy of the assessment.

For example, when preparing to transfer a head trauma patient from the acute care setting to a rehabilitation setting, the case manager will work closely with the admissions coordinator of one or more rehabilitation facilities to obtain a timely, accurate neuropsychological evaluation. This assessment can:

- determine eligibility criteria for the patient;
- assist in determining the patient's insurance coverage for treatment;
- determine the initial care plan for the patient;
- serve as a benchmark for the patient's physical, behavioral and social improvement while at the facility;
- serve as a guideline for discharge planning from the rehabilitation facility, and community re-entry.

The case manger will want to assure the following:

- The neuropsychological assessment is performed by the appropriate professional (ie, neuropsychologist) at the most appropriate intervention period, in the most timely manner possible;
- The written report is received by the case manager in a timely manner;
- The written report is shared with appropriate members of the health care team, such as the payer, the primary care physician, and other specialty physicians and therapists, who will assume treatment responsibility for the patient after discharge from the rehabilitation facility.

Psychological and neuropsychological evaluations performed during a patient's rehabilitation stay can also be excellent indicators of whether the facility can appropriately meet the needs of the patient. Other concepts and diagnostic indicators necessary to understand when considering psychological functioning include those associated with psychiatric disability. Psychiatric disability is a term that can be associated with many types of illness or injury, and is not exclusive to patients with mental health disorders. A psychiatric disability can be present in a patient with or without physical disability, and with or without co-morbid psychiatric issues. It can be chronic or acute, and even misdiagnosed, underdiagnosed, or undiagnosed by the clinical team.

CASE STUDY

Consider a workers' compensation case in which a bank teller was involved in an armed robbery. The bank teller sustained a gun shot wound to the right arm and was being treated aggressively to regain full function of his shoulder, arm, wrist, and hand. After immediate surgery collaboratively by an orthopedic surgeon and a hand surgeon, the patient was scheduled for physical and occupational therapy, pain management, and a work hardening program. However, despite aggressive management by the interdisciplinary team, the patient was nonadherent with his treatment regimen and was labeled "non-compliant". The case manager, who was a clinical social worker, was the only professional to recognize that the patient was suffering from post-traumatic stress disorder (PTSD), causing him to retreat from interactions, communication, and other "compliant" situations. Once the patient's PTSD was diagnosed, addressed, and treated, the patient was able to manage his post-acute treatment regimen. Recognizing the PTSD also allowed the case manager to request a vocational evaluation for the patient, which resulted in identifying new employment opportunities for the patient in another career, and spurred the patient's recovery period. Information on vocational evaluations will be covered in Chapter three.

Obviously, understanding psychiatric disabilities is a critical component of the case management process. It requires use of learned clinical skills and a keen awareness of the possibility for psychiatric disability among patients who may not be considered as having mental health disorders . Case managers may not be experts or even have specific experience in mental or behavioral health; however, case managers should recognize that there are a myriad of situations when psychiatric disability issues can be diagnosed, and when a silent co-morbid condition can impact a patient's physical health and overall quality of life. Some case examples include:

- a cancer patient experiencing depression;
- AIDS patient on HAART medication regimen who experiences vivid, irrational nightmares, resulting in paranoia;
- traumatic brain injury patient with perseveration, stemming from chronic obsessive compulsive disorder, exacerbated by the TBI;
- Hepatitis C patient experiencing chronic fatigue, leading to suicidal tendencies.

All case managers, regardless of practice setting, discipline, or caseload will likely work with patients and families affected by a psychiatric disability. When planning long-term goals for a depressed, suicidal patient, the case manager will assist the patient in developing more effective coping mechanisms. Other interventions, however, may not be as obvious.

This is also true when considering patients with substance use, abuse, and/or addiction. The term substance abuse can imply the stereotype patient—a drug addict or an alcoholic. These patients are often considered as having mental health disorders and dual diagnoses. In fact, many of them do require mental health treatment during a specific timeframe in their lives, or their treatment and addiction management can be lifelong. However, substance use, abuse, and/or addiction involves patients, and even co-workers in many different scenarios that are not as readily identified or understood. Examples include:

1. *Polypharmacy.* Polypharmacy is the unwanted duplication of drugs and often results when patients see multiple physicians or frequent, multiple pharmacies. Patients are also at risk for polypharmacy if they use homeopathic, supplemental, over-the-counter or herbal medicines.

Polypharmacy behavior can be unintentional by a patient, who may be seeking competitive drug pricing, or may be using various pharmacies with locations convenient to work, home, and social events. This behavior can also be intentional by a patient who is drug seeking. Fortunately, recently developed software and information technology (IT) systems have decreased this action and have enabled pharmacists to alert the ordering physician regarding potential abuses. These software and IT systems can interface with disease management systems, where pharmacy data and claims data are used to stratify health patterns and health profiles of patients. More information on disease management and data management systems will be covered in Chapters four and seven.

Software systems are also currently being utilized by some of the large retail drug chains as part of a value-added support system offered to payers. These software systems assist the pharmacists to provide valuable print education to individual patients regarding drug interactions, adherence to a drug treatment regimen, and other useful tips that are specific to the patient and the patient's prescription profile.

Case managers can assist patients who may be at-risk for polypharmacy behavior. Questions to ask the patient include:

1. Do you take five or more prescribed medications?
2. Do you take dietary supplements, vitamins, over-the-counter drugs, homeopathic remedies or herbal medicines?
3. Are you using different pharmacies to fill your prescriptions?
4. How many doctors currently provide you with prescriptions?
5. Do you take your medicines more often than once or twice a day?
6. Do you have impaired eyesight or hearing or do you live alone?

2. Polymedicine patient who sees several different physicians. This behavior prevents physicians from having knowledge of the treatment by other physicians, and from having knowledge of other prescriptions written for the patient.

Polymedicine is a behavior that can be unintentional by a patient who is unaware of the dangers of polymedicine, including conflicting treatment regimens, drug interactions, and drug overdose. Polymedicine is particularly a problem among the older generation, where it is not uncommon for a husband and wife to plan a good part of their week around various doctors' appointments. Older individuals possessing traditional Medicare plans are more likely to visit multiple physicians than are individuals in managed care insurance plans, where referrals to specialists are often required as a mechanism to thwart polymedicine behavior. Polymedicine can also be an intentional behavior by a patient who is drug seeking or treatment seeking.

3. Chronic pain patients on multiple pain drugs. One of the most common mistakes made by health care professionals is the assumption that a patient experiencing chronic pain is addicted to the medications.

Chronic pain patients often have a dependency for a pain medication regimen that allows them to tolerate their activities of daily living and lead near-normal lives. However, having dependency for pain medication is very different from having an addiction. Consider the diabetic patient, who must take daily insulin injections to maintain appropriate glucose levels. The diabetic patient is dependent upon insulin medication but is not considered addicted to the medication. Pain specialists compare the diabetic's need for insulin to the chronic pain patient's need for pain medication. Unfortunately, patients often do not receive appropriate pain management because of misguided and misunderstood concerns regarding dependency versus addiction. Chronic pain patients are often mislabeled as addicted, drug seeking, or drug abusers.[4]

Case managers must rely on their clinical skills to assist them in recognizing and appropriately managing the array of challenges stemming from the patient with substance use/abuse/addiction. As stated earlier, assessment tools and diagnostic tests are also useful. One common, effective assessment tool for the substance abuse patient is the Basis 32. The Basis 32 is a health assessment screening tool meant to assess the overall mental health of a patient, and has had particular success when used by the case manager for substance use/abuse/addiction patients. More information on the use of health assessment screening tools is covered in Chapter four.

REFERRALS

Regardless of whether the case manager's role involves the patient's physical or psychological functioning, he/she can be effective only if an appropriate referral has been made. An appropriate referral is one that is timely, fiscally responsible, and in the best interests of the patient/family being served. Over the years, health care organizations have spent countless hours and dollars to refine internal referral processes. Elaborate systems have been developed in an effort to effectively triage patients into case management, assuming that the earlier patients are identified, the better the patient can be managed in a quality, cost- effective manner.

Appropriate

The early identification of cases is essential to contain the cost of health care services as well as to improve compliance to the treatment plan.[5] Therefore, the first step in the case management process is to identify patients who will be referred to case management services. Identification of patients requiring case management services ensures that the patient is appropriate for case management interventions. Identification of patients must occur before assessment of the patient can begin. The Standards of Practice for Case Management, published by the Case Management Society of America, states that the first step in the case management process is to appraise the need for case management intervention through critical, objective evaluation of relevant data.[6]

> "The case manager will evaluate proactive triggers (such as criteria related to diagnosis, complications, or cost) to identify potential patients suitable for effective case management intervention."[7]

Timely

Computer software equipment is commonly used in larger health care organizations, such as insurance companies, hospital systems, post-acute facilities, and even in case management companies to identify potential cases suitable for timely case management intervention. Software can be programmed to flag claims exceeding a certain dollar amount per episode of illness, or to track and flag claims exceeding a certain number of hospitalizations in a given time period. Software is often used in conjunction with utilization management (UM) systems. UM reviewers in insurance companies often triage patients to case management during their precertification and concurrent review processes. More information on UM will be provided in Chapter six. Software in hospital systems may triage patients into case management, or define recommended standards for discharge planning and case management intervention. The trick is not just to determine whether referral to case management is appropriate, but to determine the optimal window of intervention to ensure quality, cost-effective outcomes.

Fiscally Responsible

Just as the mechanisms used to identify patients for case management are broad and varied, the number of referral sources are enormous. Case managers can receive referrals from integrated health care delivery systems, insurance company in-house triage systems, outside insurance adjusters, third-party administrators, acute and post-acute health care facilities, social service agencies, attorneys, employers, federal systems, other health care professionals, or directly from patients/families. Because of this, there may be great variation in how the case manager initiates intervention.

The way in which a case manager approaches a new case is greatly influenced by the referral source and the payer system.[8] Issues such as insurance policy limits, available coverage, eligibility for benefits, available funds, and other fiscal issues must be considered when determining a plan of care. Yet, it is the case manager's responsibility to exercise fiscal responsibility when accepting a referral, receiving a patient into a facility, or arranging a discharge, regardless of the pay source and whether services are covered.

Sometimes an acute care facility may have a clear financial advantage in keeping a patient; yet, the case manager knows that the patient could receive quality care in a less intensive level of service, such as a subacute facility or even in the patient's home, as explored in Chapter one. It is the case manager's responsibility to recommend discharge to the appropriate service location, regardless of financial incentives. On the other hand, a patient may have exceeded major medical benefits of the health plan but continues to require services in a health care facility. Rather than close the case, the case manager is responsible to explore/identify appropriate community services, and arrange transfer for the patient once a new plan can be implemented. In another example, the independent case manager receiving a patient referral from a payer should not accept the case if case management intervention is not appropriate or in the best interest of the patient, even if the payer source pre-approves payment for case management services.

CASE STUDY

A brain injured patient is referred to an independent case manager by his appointed guardian, who is responsible for his estate. The guardian guarantees payment of case management services using funds from the patient's estate. In the fact-gathering stage following referral, the independent case manager learns that the patient has group health insurance coverage. She contacts the benefits manager at the insurance company and discovers that the patient's group health insurance plan provides for catastrophic case management at no additional charge to the patient, and without impacting the patient's available benefits. The independent case manager then contacts the insurance company case management department and successfully transitions the patient to the appropriate in-house catastrophic case manager. The independent case manager then notifies the guardian with this information, offering to periodically monitor the case if needed, and to intervene if necessary. Although she has lost the case and many billable hours, the independent case manager has performed in a fiscally responsible manner, advocating for the best interests of the patient.

The case manager also must assume responsibility for referrals that he/she gives or implies. Case managers spend a great deal of time and energy on the planning process of the care plan. During this time, the case manager is contacting appropriate service providers, in order to ascertain the following:

- if the provider can provide the necessary scope of service in a timely, quality-based, and acceptable manner;
- what the cost will be, and whether the provider's services and fees are a covered benefit under the patient's insurance plan or pay source;
- whether the provider possesses the appropriate accreditation, licensure, and levels of staff competency as deemed appropriate by the case manager and/or the payer to meet the needs of the patient.

Once the case manager has completed this fact-finding portion of the planning phase and is ready to make referrals to appropriate service providers, the case manager will implement the care plan. The provider of service will usually require a signed contract between the provider and the payer or the payer's duly appointed representative. The case manager must be aware that in a stated contract from the provider, it is implied that the provider will be paid for the services rendered. Therefore, it is very important that the case manager maintain fiscal responsibility in choosing, implementing, and coordinating referrals with service providers. Additional information on provider relationships is covered in Chapter ten.

CONSULTATION

Once the referral process is completed, the case manager will employ his/her clinical skills in a comprehensive fact-finding assessment process. It is the case manager's responsibility to conduct a thorough and objective evaluation of the patient's current status, including medical, financial, psychological, social, and vocational aspects. Obviously, to accomplish this, the case manager will need to collaborate with the family, payer, and employer (if any). The case manager will also need to consult with several different members of the health care team.

Consultation is the act of conferring with another individual in order to gain an opinion or advice. One individual usually consults with another individual because the second person is considered an expert who can give professional advice or services. Consultation is a large part of the fact-finding and assessment stage in case management. However, consultation with other members of the health care team continues throughout all phases of the case management process and is one of the defining factors in creating a holistic, objective, and effective plan of care.

Physician

The physician is the key decision maker regarding the patient's treatment plan and is, therefore, often the most important consultant to the clinical case manager. While the physician develops an ongoing treatment plan, the case manager develops an ongoing care plan. Together they can have an extraordinary, positive impact on the holistic wellness and health of a patient. Yet, most case managers are not entirely comfortable dealing with physicians, and some will even avoid speaking to the physician, which can certainly compromise health care outcomes for the patient.

While case managers and physicians alike consider patient advocacy as their primary responsibility, historically these two professionals have not collaborated effectively to provide the best patient advocacy possible. Much of the problem stems from lack of understanding and initiative from both sides regarding the importance of each to the patient's health care outcomes. The following role depictions offered by each side can stymie professional collaboration between physicians and case managers.

Another fundamental difference is the approach in practice of each professional. Physicians have traditionally been autocratic, assuming final, sole responsibility legally and ethically for care of the patient. Case managers by their very processes are team-oriented and accustomed to collaboration. Therefore, it is in the best interest of the case manager—and the patient—for the case manager to assume a lead role in developing a relationship with the patient's physician.

Physician's View Point	Case Manager's View Point
The physician may view the case manager as undermining the doctor-patient relationship.	The case manager may view the physician as focusing on biological improvement without regard to quality of life.
The physician may believe the case manager rations health care.	The case manager may believe the physician over-utilizes health care resources.
The physician believes he/she can best communicate, and has the trust of the patient.	The case manager believes he/she can best communicate and has the trust of the patient.
The physician feels the case manager does not understand disease progression or symptom management.	The case manager feels the physician does not recognize viable options and alternatives in disease and symptom management.
The physician believes the case manager encourages patients to seek inappropriate resources and venues for health information.	The case manager believes the physician does not adequately use information technology or evidence-based practices, such as algorithms and clinical pathways, in treatment decisions.

One way to enhance the working relationship between the case manager and the physician is to assure the physician that findings, concerns, and suggestions will be presented for review. In other words, the case manager will review and consider implementation of a suggestion by the physician, while the case manager will also present appropriate recommendations, concerns, and findings to the physician, which can be suggested by any member of the health care team, including the patient. It is important to assure the physician that he/she will be updated on the patient's status on a continuous basis. However, the case manager must be sensitive to how often updates should occur—providing daily reports to the physician's staff is usually unnecessary and inappropriate, just as holding information for extended periods of time between communications is inappropriate.

A case manager who has developed a positive relationship with a physician is in a much more advantageous position to "make things happen" for the patient. These could include:

- suggesting potential alternatives to the treatment plan that can enhance quality and lower costs;
- arranging out-of-benefit resources covered by the payer, based on a letter of medical necessity from the physician and supportive documentation;
- initiating a discussion between the payer's medical director and the patient's physician, which results in better care for the patient;
- enlisting the physician in problem solving on a current, or a future, difficult case;
- using the physician as an informational resource or an actual referral source for other cases.

A White Paper exploring best practices in physician and case manager collaboration was co-sponsored by CMSA and the authors of this book in 2003, following a national summit of key opinion leaders—medical directors of health plans, physicians in private practice, nurse case managers in payer and provider settings—which convened in April 2003. The *Consensus Paper of the 2003 Physician and Case Management Summit: Exploring Best Practices in Physician and Case Management Collaboration to Improve Patient Care* provides barriers and facilitators to effective collaboration between physicians and case managers. (See Table 1 and Table 2.)

Pharmacist

Of course, there are other members of the health care team who are also important consultants to the effective case manager—among them, the pharmacist. Several years ago, teaching institutions began encouraging pharmacists to complete morning rounds with physicians in acute care settings. The in-

---

Table 1: Barriers to Effective Collaboration Between Physicians and Case Managers

1. Lack of resources among physicians to achieve case management integration.
2. Lack of time among physicians to understand and learn about case management.
3. Lack of scientific evidence to support the value of case management.
4. Poor financial incentives among physicians to support case management processes.
5. Physician resistance to change.
6. Lack of aligned incentives among physicians, case managers and patients served.
7. Systems variability.
8. Multiple case management standards and guidelines.
9. No uniformity in certification or training among case managers.
10. Education silos between physician and case manager academia.
11. Fragmentation of communication in the current health care system.
12. Legal and regulatory hurdles.
13. Limited knowledge by physicians of how to access and use of case managers.
14. Misunderstanding by physicians of the role of the case manager in multiple settings.
15. Lack of consumer awareness of case management.

Adapted from Moreo K. Consensus Paper of the 2003 Physician and Case Management Summit. 2003: CMSA and PRIME

Table 2: Facilitators to Effective Collaboration Between Physicians and Case Managers

1. Effective systems-based models for communication and collaboration among the care coordination team
2. Studies that produce evidence-based, outcomes-driven case management data
3. Recognition of the heterogeneity of case management
4. Standardization of education, training in case management
5. Standardization of case management definitions among certifying and accreditation bodies
6. Leadership-supported information technology to decrease case management fragmentation
7. Consumer based and physician based education about case management; empowering patients when and how to access case management services
8. Circulate CMSA Standards of Practice for Case Management and other standards available
9. Trust-building techniques between physicians and case managers
10. Models and organizations that promote accountability in case management
11. Skills-building training of case managers to effectively/appropriately challenge decisions by the physician that are not in the patient's best interest
12. Financial enumeration to physicians for collaboration with case managers

Adapted from Moreo K. Consensus Paper of the 2003 Physician and Case Management Summit. 2003: CMSA and PRIME.

creased role that pharmacy and drug management play in health care delivery make it essential for the case manager to consult regularly with pharmacists. Biological and technological advances in medicine continue to escalate the use of medications in health care. With this comes an increase in the incidence of drug interactions, drug sensitivity, drug overdose, and polypharmacy. As noted earlier in this chapter, polypharmacy is a critical problem among many patients, and pharmacists are in a key position to curb or eliminate this potentially dangerous situation.

Pharmacists can be consulted to assist the case manager in understanding the various prescribing habits of physicians, or to strategize an approach to the patient's physician when attempting to suggest a potential alternative drug intervention. Pharmacists can be an excellent resource for those cases where the patient is prescribed a battery of drugs, and the case manager is engaged in educating the patient, which requires a knowledge of drugs' indications, side effects, etc. Pharmacists can be a great ally when the case manager is dealing with a noncompliant or nonadherent patient. They can assist in monitoring the patient's medication compliance, as well as offer education and support to the patient to increase compliance. Pharmacists can also be an excellent source of information for the patient, and be a vital link in establishing a relationship with the patient that is built upon trust.

Nurse

Whether or not the case manager is a nurse, he/she should communicate as a clinician when consulting with a nurse. As highly skilled clinicians, nurses can be excellent consultants and good sources of information for the case manager. Staff nurses are reliable historians when dealing with a patient in an acute care setting, rehabilitation facility, or long-term care facility. They can report on a patient's physical, mental and behavioral status; they can provide insight into family dynamics; they can assess the patient's ongoing responsiveness to the treatment plan; and, like the case manager, they are trained to view the patient holistically, making them a valuable resource to the clinical case manager. Often, bedside nurses are caring for the patient because of their expertise in the patient's particular disease process or injury. Therefore, they are also excellent sources of information pertaining to the patient's diagnosis and prognosis.

Nutritionist

The nutritionist can also be a valuable source of information regarding the patient's nutritional status. This is particularly true in cases where nutritional intake profoundly affects the patient's disease process, such as diabetes, coronary artery disease, cancer, Crohn's disease, ulcerative colitis, malabsorption, and metabolic disorders. The diabetic patient is most successful with therapeutic intervention when he/she can be educated about dietary planning in accordance with the American Diabetes Association (ADA). The ADA recommends specific caloric guidelines for daily meal planning of diabetics: 60% complex carbohydrates; 12%–15% protein; 20%–25% fat. Nutritionists can be invaluable in the initial education, as well as the continuing education of diabetic patients, to ensure their compliance with a dietary regimen.

Nutritionists are excellent resource persons in those cases where nutrition may not be as evident. One example is the assistance of a nutritionist for a patient with AIDS. The nutritionist can track dietary deficiencies of the patient with AIDS, with goals of preventing wasting and maximizing energy levels. The nutritionist will assist the case manager to develop action steps, and then promote buy-in from the patient to maximize effectiveness. Appropriate action steps include intervening with nutritional supplements as soon as the patient with AIDS has lost 10% of body weight, or teaching the patient simple meal planning to maximize effective dietary intake while minimizing energy spent by the patient.

Another example involves the nutritionist as a consultant on a psychiatric disability case. When patients are bulimic or anorexic, it is easy to determine the need for a nutritional consult. However, consider the bipolar patient who continues to be hyperactive and to lose weight at an alarming pace. The case manager notices that the family encourages the patient to eat small, frequent meals that can be carried, in order to comply with the patient's hyperactivity. The case manager consults a nutritionist to work with the patient and the family. The patient and family are educated about mealtime needs. The patient is provided a quiet, comfortable and attractive place in which to sit down to eat meals.

Nutritionists are also effective consultants when managing patients with cancer. Many oncology patients on chemotherapy develop anemia and anemia-related fatigue. Nutritional interventions that are essential to the plan of care and that can be supported by a nutritionist include:

- monitoring the treatment plan to ensure that the patient is prescribed anti-emetics prior to chemotherapy treatments;
- monitoring B-12 and folic acid intake to minimize anemia resulting from chemotherapy-induced immunosuppression;
- providing teaching and training for low-maintenance meal preparation and high-energy food sources, to minimize the fatigue and anemia;
- providing teaching and training to enhance the sensory pleasure of meals, to combat nausea, and to enhance food intake.[10]

Each of the foregoing examples demonstrates opportunities for dieticians and nutritional experts to specialize in case management. In population health models where nutrition is a primary focus to maintain wellness—such as in the diabetic population—licensed, trained dieticians often assume the role of the case manager. This is because the dietician has special training and expertise that allows the professional to effectively educate patients and even positively modify patient behaviors.

Physical Therapist and Occupational Therapist

As ancillary professionals, physical therapists (PTs) and occupational therapists (OTs) are excellent resources to the case manager, or can assume specialty case management roles. Like nutritionists, PTs and OTs possess specific knowledge and skills pertinent to a patient's disease process and prognosis. Like nurses, PTs and OTs can provide clinical expertise and historical "bedside" information to the case manager that is invaluable when developing, implementing, and monitoring a plan of care. Many OTs and PTs are excellent case managers. Most PTs and OTs are accustomed to, and comfortable with, consulting case managers. Many are accustomed to participating with case managers in the acute-care and post-acute care settings in periodic team staffings, where each member of the inter-disciplinary team provides a brief update on the patient's progress.

PTs and OTs enhance and maximize the patient's functional status through one-on-one training, exercise, and behavior modification. They fully understand functional capacity, and are prepared to successfully interact with the patient/family. Experienced case managers report instances when the patient shared pertinent, valuable information only with the PT or OT. Successful PTs and OTs develop trusting relationships with their patients, and are therefore able to encourage their patients to perform exercise and treatment regimens that may painful but are necessary to achieve wellness.

Case managers can consult with PTs and OTs to learn more about the behavioral aspects of the patient and important family dynamics. OTs comprehensively assess the home environment regarding function and safety. Hospital discharge planners use OTs to complete home evaluations, where they examine the need for necessary changes, such as structural modifications, improved lighting, or removal of hazardous elements, ie, throw rugs, exposed electrical cords, high cabinets, or slippery tile. As patients are being discharged to home much earlier from hospitals, with more complex needs, the condition of the home environment becomes a critical factor in safe discharge planning. More information on home assessments to promote safe discharges is covered in Chapter five.

Social Worker

Whether or not the case manager is a social worker, he/she should regularly consult with a social worker, particularly when dealing with fragile populations, psychosocial issues, difficult family dynamics, or financial constraints that affect a patient. Social workers are excellent sources of information for the case manager.

A particular strength of social workers is that of resource management. They are usually well versed in available community resources that can be used when payer benefits are not available for a needed service or product. Social workers are experienced at mobilizing financial resources for eligible patients, such as Medicaid, vocational rehabilitation, social security disability income, or social service state-funded programs. They implement application processes early, familiar with the denials and long wait-lists often associated with these resources. Social workers are such a critical component in the case management process that many health care delivery systems engage social workers to interface with medical case managers, usually nurses, in a team case management approach.

COLLABORATION

Equally important to consultation in the case management process, is collaboration. Collaboration is listed as a standard of performance in the CMSA Standards of Practice for Case Management[11], and is discussed briefly in Chapter 1. It is the common thread that weaves together assessment, planning, implementation, coordination, interaction, monitoring and evaluation. Collaboration is the glue that binds all processes of case management together.

When the case manager consults with various health care professionals as defined earlier in this chapter, he/she is collaborating peer-to-peer to effect positive change for the patient and family. When the telephonic case manager is contacting all providers in a patient's care plan to ascertain progress and identify problems, he/she is collaborating peer-to-peer to effect positive change. When the acute-care case manager talks quietly with the family to relieve their anxiety about a loved one's failing health status, he/she is collaborating person-to-person to effect positive change. Collaboration occurs so dynamically in case management that it often goes unrecognized.

Client/Family

Collaboration with the patient/family is a fundamental role of the case manager. The case manager actively engages the patient and the family in the care plan by collaborating to maximize health care outcomes. Engaging the patient and family as active participants includes:

- seeking their input, support, and buy-in to the dynamic plan of care, including any changes to the care plan;

- nurturing their strength as a family unit, encouraging their mutual involvement, and respecting their differences;
- assisting them to understand and to manage the complex health issues new to them;
- initiating an individualized approach to the care plan that is suited to their culture, beliefs, and wishes.

Collaborating with the patient/family is a component of family-centered case management, recognizing that the family is our most important basic social institution, and plays the preeminent role in the case and in nurturing its members.[12] Family-centered case management supports families who are suddenly thrown into the role of caregiver, and assists them in their commitment to providing for the well-being of their ill or injured member. When the case manager practices family-centered case management, he/she enables the family to become more competent and independent in meeting their needs, by providing opportunities for their participation.

Interdisciplinary Team

In collaborating with the patient and family, the case manager facilitates collaboration between the patient/family and the interdisciplinary team, so that the patient/family is viewed by all members of the health care team as being at the center of care. Further, the case manager collaborates effectively and in a timely manner, directly with members of the interdisciplinary team.

Collaboration occurs in a variety of ways and through a variety of venues—by 1) ongoing one-on-one telephone communication or shared teleconference calls; 2) providing written narrative reports to all parties, 3) sharing charting/documentation that is e-mailed for review and group comment, and 4) face-to-face meetings. Confidentiality issues regarding the patient's right to privacy arise with each of these communication methods, and the case manager must be aware of policies and procedures in the workplace that address who, what, when, and how a patient's medical information will be shared. Patient confidentiality and security are addressed in Chapter ten.

Acute-care case managers have the greatest advantage in collaborating with the interdisciplinary team, if they engage in regularly scheduled team staffings. Staff meetings engage all members of the health care team in a brief sharing of information about the patient's response to treatment, and includes the patient/family in the staff meetings. Usually, the case manager is the team leader, serving as a facilitator, and ensuring that information is exchanged collaboratively, in a timely manner.

Employer

In workers' compensation or disability insurance cases, the employer is a key individual for case manager collaboration regarding the patient's plan of care. A main goal of workers' compensation is to return the injured/ill employee to gainful employment. The case manager may need to collaborate with the employer, to determine such issues as whether accommodations can be made for a patient recovering from an illness or injury; whether a patient can return to work on a part-time or limited-hours basis; whether there is a job for the employee to return to after an extended illness; or whether a patient's job description can be modified based on health-related limitations.

Even if the case is not related to workers' compensation, the patient's employer can be an important person to collaborate with regarding the patient's treatment plan. Patient confidentiality must be maintained, but the case manager can talk with the employer to suggest supportive measures that may be taken to assist the patient during a long illness/injury or recovery period. These measures may include requesting uplifting telephone calls or visits to the patient by co-workers; or contact with the patient by the employer to allay any fears of job loss or of increased workload.

Payer

Collaboration between the case manager and the payer is imperative. Even when case managers work directly for the payer, internal formal communication and collaboration are required as part of the case manager's responsibilities. When the case manager does not work for the payer, he/she is still responsible to collaborate effectively and efficiently with the payer in order to ensure adequate and timely health care coverage.

Payers maintain that external case managers are expected to be the "eyes and ears" of the payer. Payers report frustration when a plan member is hospitalized beyond expected days, and the payer cannot obtain sufficient information from the facility to explain the need for the extended hospitalization. Similarly, acute- care case managers report frustration when they seek authorization by the payer for services required by the patient, and cannot reach the payer, or arrange a collaborative discussion. Obviously, developing and maintaining a collaborative relationship between the case manager and the payer is a win-win goal for both sides.

EDUCATION

Education is the final point to be discussed when considering clinical practice in case management. Clinical case managers from all practice settings, regardless of discipline, job title, or level of experience agree that education of the patient/family/caregiver is an essential part of the case manager's clinical practice. An experienced case manager will seize every communication opportunity with the patient, family and/or caregiver to educate them regarding disease process, prognosis, symptom management, self-care opportunities, wellness/prevention strategies, and other pertinent topics to enhance health care outcomes.

Effective education is continuous, reinforced at every opportunity, is non-judgmental, objective, and free of personal opinion. Topics for education of patients, families, and caregivers by the case manager are broad and diverse, including medication management and side effects, diet, clinical tasks to perform for self-care, disease progression and prognosis, treatment information to promote informed decision-making, benefits coverage, prevention or elimination of environmental hazards, and end-of-life decisions.

Delivery Techniques

As the case manager educates, reinforces, and evaluates ongoing educational needs/techniques, he/she is in a unique position to monitor the patient's compliance with treatment and medication regimens; to monitor the need for more effective education, or education by other specialty health care professionals; and to evaluate the need for attendant care, a home health nurse, or a language interpreter during education sessions. The case manager can identify the need for alternative interactions, such as an unplanned visit to the physician's office, a telephone call with the patient's bank or financial advisor, and the need for spiritual guidance and religious support.

All of these identifiers, triggers, and troubleshooting opportunities are possible only when the case manager is an effective observer. Effective education is based on effective delivery of the message, which includes awareness of one's body language, facial expressions, personal feelings and emotions, and in exercising tact and diplomacy, including using the essential skill of listening. As an educator, the case manager must be sensitive to the needs of the patient, family, and/or caregiver, and must use sensitive listening skills to actively engage others in the process. Listening is as important a part of education as speaking. As the case manager continues to learn diverse methods of education, he/she becomes a master of the art.

Education by the case manager can also occur with other individuals involved in the health care continuum, such as other members of the healthcare team, the employer, and the payer. The case manager is often in a position to educate other members of the healthcare team and the payer regarding changes in the patient's status, resources that may be available, alternatives to treatment, and issues pertaining to the patient/family that may be pertinent to expected outcomes, such as family dynamics or cultural issues. In a workers' compensation setting, the case manager often communicates with the employer, offering education that can assist in a successful return-to-work for the employee. Information on education of the employer is covered in Chapter three.

Application of Clinical Practice

The following section is intended to offer disease-specific and injury-specific care plan goals for some of the complex, high-cost conditions that case managers are often called upon to manage. As stated earlier in this chapter, many clinical case managers specialize in these conditions, but often it is the generalist case manager who is coordinating care for a complex patient. Having core knowledge regarding disease-specific and injury-specific goals that would typically be included in each of the presented disease or injury processes is essential for the case manager to understand. Written examinations traditionally test the case manager's knowledge of complex, high-cost diseases and injuries, so this becomes an important area for case managers to review when preparing for certification. Overall, the goal that case managers strive to achieve when working with complex patients, is to provide effective health management that enables patients to maintain an optimal quality of life. The true test of case managers' success is the transfer of knowledge and accountability regarding the patients' and families' needs in a manner that promotes optimal health and wellness.

HIV/AIDS

Much progress has been made in the treatment of patients diagnosed with HIV/AIDS. The development of protease inhibitors and other life-sustaining drugs has shifted the view on HIV/AIDS as a chronic condition that can be managed, rather than a terminal illness. Case managers who work with HIV/AIDS patients must continue to educate patients regarding the importance of compliance to treatment, and empower them to take responsibility for their care. Nutritional management, exercise, proper rest, and spiritual awareness are all important aspects for the case manager to incorporate into plans of care, and to monitor to ensure that the patient is on a steady course. Patients need to understand outcomes of various lab tests that are performed routinely to follow these aspects of the disease.

For example, Mary, a newly diagnosed patient and mother of two, was recently prescribed HAART (Highly Active Antiretroviral Therapy) following a hospitalization for pneumocystis carinii. Mary is told to call the case manager at the primary care clinic to obtain monthly results of her lab work. The case manager assigned to follow Mary explains that the results of the lab work are very good. The case manager explained that Mary's CD4+ count is 655, indicating that Mary's immune system is functioning and able to fight infection. Another positive sign is that Mary's viral load is below detectable levels. The case manager informs Mary that her hemoglobin and hematocrit dropped since her discharge from the hospital. She explains that this was expected, since the protease inhibitors she is taking to control the disease, suppress the bone marrow, causing hematopoiesis to decline. The case manager advises Mary to report immediately any signs or symptoms of fatigue. In order to effectively monitor this, the case manager asks Mary to keep a record of how she is doing with regard to her activities of daily living (ADLs). The case manager explains that if Mary's hemoglobin continues to drop, she will experience a decrease in her ability to perform normal activities. Repeat labs will be done in another month to closely monitor the levels. If the hemoglobin and hematocrit level drop below a certain level, or if Mary experiences difficulty with her ADLs, a preventive medication may be given that will stimulate and maintain a consistent production of erythropoetin, to assist the body in producing more red blood cells. The case manager explains that if this is not done proactively, and the hemoglobin and hematocrit continue to decrease, Mary may need to be admitted to the hospital to receive a blood transfusion. Mary tells the case manager she has spent enough time in the hospital and will do whatever it takes to stay healthy so she can continue to work.

The case manager asks Mary if she is taking her medications as prescribed. Mary relates that taking so many pills is very difficult, but she understands the importance of taking them. She relays her medication routine to the case manager. Mary also mentions that she had lost a few pounds due to nausea and inability to eat. The case manager notes that the last weight taken was adequate, but that on the next visit the patient should again be weighed. She realizes that if a patient with HIV/AIDS drops more than ten percent of this/her body weight, nutritional supplements are usually initiated. The case manager tells Mary that she is doing well and to keep up the good work. She tells Mary she will send her a card with her next appointment date, but to feel free to call her if any problems arise.

By having close contact with the patient, the case manager can alert the physician and the health care team of any problems before serious complications occur. The goal is to keep the patient as healthy as possible, and to identify problems early so that interventions can be put into place. By providing education regarding complications of the disease process and informing the patient about her results, the case manager is allowing the patient to take an active role in her own care.

Brain Injury

Traumatic brain injury (TBI) usually occurs as the result of an auto accident, a fall, or some other trauma. Those who suffer from a TBI may experience complications that vary depending upon what area of the brain sustained the injury and how serious the blow to the skull is. Case managers should be aware of the anatomy of the brain and the functions that are associated with each lobe. For example, those with frontal lobe injuries may experience deficits in activities involving planning, organizing, and problem solving. They can have poor attention span and personality changes. Those with occipital lobe injuries can experience visual problems because the optic nerve is in this lobe. Temporal lobe injuries may cause deficits in the differentiation of smell and sound, short-term memory loss, and inability to process new information. The parietal lobe has two lobes, one on either side of the brain. Injury to the right lobe can cause visual-spatial deficits, or difficulty negotiating new or familiar places. Damage to the left lobe can cause difficulties with the written or spoken language. Understanding the various functions of each lobe allows the case manager to better understand how to develop a plan of care for the patient.

Initially, the patient may seem fine after an accident. The patient will be discharged from the ED following a brief loss of consciousness. Detailed head injury instructions should be given to someone other than the patient who will be responsible to observe the patient for a few hours after the injury in case any problems arise. Instructions are given to have the patient return immediately if any signs of confusion or memory loss occur. The emergency department staff evaluates each suspected TBI patient's mental status on arrival by means of the Glasgow Coma Scale to establish a baseline of cognitive and physical functioning. The Glasgow Coma Scale was reviewed in Chapter two. A patient who is awake and alert, is able to respond to voice commands, and to move all extremities will receive a high score of 15. Lower scores can indicate a problem in cognitive functioning. The following case example demonstrates a case manager's interventions for a TBI patient.

Late one day, the ED case manager is called to obtain authorization to admit a 17-year-old high school basketball player who was seen earlier in the day after an injury he sustained when practicing. In reviewing the chart, she notes that his coach had brought him to the ED after he fell and hit the back of his head on the gym floor. The patient was examined and discharged to the boy's father. A head injury instruction sheet had been reviewed with the father by the ED nurse.

Later in the day, when his mother came home, she noticed that her son was not making sense when she spoke to him, appeared drowsy, and fell when getting out of bed to go to the bathroom. The case manager notes that the patient had been discharged with a diagnosis of syncope after a fall. The physical exam on discharge showed that the patient could walk, and was aware and alert. The Glasgow score was 15. The report from the CAT scan was also normal. The second ED chart includes a second CAT, which notes a large bleed in the occipital area of the brain. A second Glasgow score of 10 provides a significant change from the first Glasgow, indicating a moderate deficit. The ED physician documented that the patient has blurry vision, which would be consistent with a hematoma causing pressure on the optic nerve. The ED physician refers the patient to the neurosurgeon on call. The patient is admitted to the intensive care unit for close observation. The neurosurgeon gives orders for the patient to be started on Dilantin™ to prevent a seizure, and requests that neurologic checks be performed every hour for two hours, then every four hours for 24 hours.

The ED case manager calls the acute care case manager covering the ICU and notifies him of the admission. He states that he will meet the family in the waiting room and inform them of the treatment plan in the unit. Upon meeting with the family, the acute care case manager discovers that they have many questions and are very worried. The case manager reassures them that their son is in good hands. He explains his role and encourages them to address any questions. The father states he wants to make sure their HMO is notified of the admission. The case manager explains how this is always done and that he will work closely with the HMO case manager to ensure that they are kept informed.

Meanwhile, the ED case manager calls the HMO utilization management department. She provides clinical and diagnostic information along with the treatment plan of the neurosurgeon. The plan is to observe the patient in order to see if the hematoma resolves, then transfer the patient to acute rehabilitation in order to address cognitive deficits. The HMO UM specialist informs the ED case manager that once the patient is stabilized, they should make arrangements with an acute rehabilitation center in the network to address the patient's needs. The UM specialist requests that a concurrent review be reported in two days. The ED case manager charts the results of the phone call and notifies the ICU case manager of the request for a concurrent review.

During rounds the next day, the ICU case manager learns from the hospitalist covering the ICU that the patient is doing better. The latest CAT scan shows that the hematoma is resolving, and the patient is less confused. The neurosurgeon signs off on the case, since surgery is not needed, and a neurologist will follow the case. The plan at this time is to begin the discharge process to an acute rehabilitation center.

The case manager calls a rehabilitation center in the patient's HMO network and requests an onsite evaluation to see if the patient meets criteria to be transferred. Later in the day, the admissions coordinator for the rehabilitation center calls and states they will accept the patient. The plan of care has been submitted to the HMO UM department, and approval has been received for the transfer. The ICU case manager speaks with the parents to obtain their approval for the transfer. He explains that the transfer is a positive sign, and that their son is going to a facility specializing in treating cognitive deficits their son is experiencing. Authorization from the parents is received, and the case manager arranges transportation with the rehabilitation facility. He also ensures that the patient's chart is copied, and that the hospitalist documents his update on the patient with the physiatrist at the receiving facility.

When the patient is successfully transferred to the rehabilitation center, an interdisciplinary health care team evaluates the patient and develops an individualized plan of care. The physiatrist speaks with the parents to give them an overview of what to expect now that their son is in a rehabilitation setting. At the same time, the rehabilitation case manager assigned to the patient receives a telephone call from the ICU case manager, requesting an update on the patient. Information is provided to the ICU case manager, who documents the follow-up phone call in the patient's hospital record.

When the team has developed the plan of care and identified the goals to be achieved, the rehabilitation case manager contacts the HMO to give an update on the team's findings and goals. The expected length of stay is four weeks. The managed care case manager now assigned to the case states she can authorize two weeks, and then re-evaluate the need for further inpatient care. She requests that a concurrent review be provided in ten days.

Over the next week, the patient's condition improves. Some behavioral problems remain, and his short-term memory is not normal, but he is able to follow commands and is independent in his ADLs. A team staffing is held, and the team recommends that the patient continue rehabilitation for another two weeks to monitor changes in the cognitive deficits. If this is not possible, a transfer to the outpatient day program is recommended as an alternative plan. The rehabilitation case manager realizes that the ability of the boy's parents to transport him to and from the outpatient clinic, and their willingness to bring him home with short-term cognitive impairments, will need to be explored with the family if this alternative plan is initiated.

The team suggests involving the parents in ongoing rehabilitation at this time, so they can obtain training on how to manage the patient once home. The rehabilitation case manager informs the team that she has placed a call to the principal at the boy's high school to determine whether they have any resources to assist the boy in transitioning back to normal school activities. She will also provide information to the parents on TBI support groups in the community.

As demonstrated in this unfolding story, the plan of care for the TBI patient in just the first week extends over three settings—the ED, the ICU and the rehabilitation hospital. This case study indicates how four case managers are each integral to moving the patient smoothly through the care continuum. Issues of authorization and proactive planning are addressed at the beginning to avoid delays in care of the patient. The challenges of managed care coverage are dealt with in an appropriate manner, and the patient and family are central to the process. Each case manager is able to perform his/her role because each has knowledge of TBI and the expected challenges that these patients present.

Spinal Cord Injury

In addition to traumatic brain injury, spinal cord injury (SCI) usually results from accidents or risky behavior. Case managers need to have a thorough understanding of the anatomy of the spine and defects which occur according to the level of injury to the spine. Anatomy shortcuts that can assist case managers include:

- Injuries to the spine at C3 or higher require ventilator support.
- Injuries at T6 and higher require education for patients and caregivers about autonomic dysreflexia. Autonomic dysreflexia is a life-threatening emergency condition that presents with a pounding headache, profuse sweating, a markedly elevated B/P, and bradycardia. The cause results from a noxious stimulus that is not transmitted properly by the brain, due to an interruption in the autonomic nervous system because of the injury. Conditions that commonly cause autonomic dysreflexia include a full bladder, fecal impaction, or tight, restrictive clothing. Immediate interventions include sitting the patient up; loosening any tight clothing, and a quick check to see if the bladder is distended or if there is a fecal impaction. Straight-catheterization or fecal removal is required if these conditions are found. Medication is sometimes given to resolve high blood pressure. Family members or other key people at work and school need to be aware of this complication, so that the patient can receive immediate attention.
- Lumbar spine injuries generally result in paraplegia.
- Sacral spine injuries generally result in the need for assistive devices when ambulating, such as a cane, walker, or braces.

As part of the rehabilitation process, the SCI patient and family should be taught how to provide care that will prevent common complications to the skin, bladder and bowel. Patients should learn how to inspect their skin to recognize early signs of skin breakdown caused by immobility. Physical therapists teach the patient the importance of shifting weight while in a wheelchair or lying in bed. Depending on the level of injury, the patient learns how to self-catheterize to empty the bladder. During this time, the rehabilitation nurse instructs the patient to examine urine for cloudiness and smell to detect early signs of bladder infection. Adequate fluid intake is important for the kidneys to filter impurities and prevent renal calculi from forming. A bowel program is taught to promote regular bowel movements. These patients are prone to muscle spasms, so stretching exercises are included in the plan of care. Patients learn the importance of working with a primary care physician, who can proactively assess new or ongoing medical complications.

As rehabilitation progresses, the health care team and the case manager recommend appropriate equipment and assistive devices to assist the patient with ADLs. Likely, the patient's home and automobile will be modified to provide optimal independence. The rehabilitation case manager collaborates with the managed care case manager to decide which providers are most suitable for equipment, supplies, and adaptations. The case manager supplies the patient with available community resources. Many communities have recreational programs for spinal cord patients, such as sailing lessons or wheelchair basketball.

The goal of spinal cord rehabilitation programs is to empower the patient to learn about the injury and comorbid conditions, to prevent complications, and to achieve maximum independence and quality of life. Patients may receive financial settlements if the injury is a result of an accident. As discussed in Chapter three, a life-care plan should be developed to research, assess, and report the present and future needs are for an individual patient, including costs over the lifetime. This knowledge enables the patient and/or the payer to plan financial viability for medical, social, psychological, and situational activities over the course of the patient's life.

Low Back Pain

The goal for the patient with chronic low back pain is to assess the level and cause of the pain, to work with an interdisciplinary team to develop a plan of care to treat the pain, and to encourage the patient to participate in life-long rehabilitation to maintain function and control pain. Case managers who work with patients having catastrophic illnesses and injuries may not view low back pain as a high priority. Yet, low back pain contributes to high medical costs and lost productivity costs, since many patients with low back pain are unable to work or attend school.

The key to effective pain management is to identify those patients who are not benefiting from conservative therapy, and to refer them to a specialist who can evaluate the patient's pain, properly diagnosis its cause, and devise a comprehensive plan for pain management.

Transplant Patient

Patients with organ failure compose another segment of the population with challenging disease processes that have high costs, and who often require lifelong medical care. Case managers are challenged when working with these patients and their families to ensure that they are well educated to make informed decisions that will impact care over time.

Patients need supportive care while waiting to receive an organ. Complications must be addressed in a timely manner to ensure that the patient is in the best physical and mental condition when an organ becomes available. The patient and family require a great deal of emotional support during the waiting period to assist them to cope with a failing body system.

If an organ becomes available and the patient is able to be transplanted, discharge plans must include short-term and long-term goals. The case manager is responsible for selecting a company to supply lifelong medications, negotiate costs, and arrange delivery mechanisms to support patient adherence. Patients and family members need to know about signs and symptoms of organ rejection. If patients do not receive organs in time, supportive care is provided to the patient and family to help them support the patient and to make end-of-life decisions.

Oncology

Working with patients who are diagnosed with cancer, regardless of age, is a challenge for case managers who manage the numerous resources that this population needs to access. The primary goals in cancer care are prevention, early identification of the disease process, appropriate treatments to eliminate or control the spread of cancer, and/or palliative care. It is very easy to overuse services when coordinating care for a cancer patient. Case managers who work with oncology patients can avoid overuse of services by educating the patient about side effects of treatments and aggressively managing these. The case manager is responsible to teach the patient and family, and to support them to develop and use coping skills. Centers of excellence in oncology and programs that offer clinical trials for specific cancers are excellent resources for the patient and family.

High Risk Pregnancy

Many chronic conditions that children have are congenital defects related to premature births. Early identification of women who are at risk for premature birth that could result in congenital problems is important to prevent or minimize defects that might result from prematurity. Case mangers in this field can work to ensure that resources are used appropriately to provide assistance to patients in least-restrictive settings. Creative care plans are recommended that may include out-of-benefit services if the savings produced can outweigh costs. The following case study demonstrates this point.

Pat is a 42-year-old mother of one child who is pregnant with twins. She had an uneventful pregnancy until 32 weeks' gestation when she began to spot. She saw her doctor who advised hospital admission to delay delivery. The doctor informs the patient that the goal is to bring her as close to 40 weeks' gestation as possible. He believes that she cannot rest at home with an active three-year-old. The managed care case manager receives a request for hospital admission, and calls the woman to discuss options. She realizes that the mother is distraught about having to be in the hospital for as long as eight weeks. She says that her husband is able to care for the child at night, but works during the day. The case manager explores day care, but the woman says that they cannot afford a day-care program. Another option is to place a home-care aide in the home to care for the child during the day, which allows the child to stay in the home environment.

Pat likes this plan, but doesn't know whether the insurance company pays for a babysitter. The case manager learns that this is not a covered benefit. However, if the physician will agree to home-based bed rest for Pat, this may be an alternative that can be approved by the obstetrician. The managed care organization's medical director agrees to the plan because of the significant savings possible to the plan. Health insurance will cover the cost of home monitoring equipment and the home care nurse, who will monitor the patient telephonically. Also included is the cost of an aide for up to four hours a day to assist with child care.

The case manager makes arrangements for a fetal monitor, the home health aide, and for Pat's mother to come every afternoon to care for the 3 year old until Pat's husband returns from work.

The outcome of this case study is that Pat did well and delivered twins at 39 weeks' gestation. Both babies were born with Apgar scores of 8/10. This case is an example of how a case manager organizes a creative plan of care to meet the needs of the patient. The savings generated from this case were significant, since hospitalization costs were avoided for 49 days.

When children are born prematurely, the case manager will usually open a new case, since there are now two patients who need to be managed—mother and baby. Providing support to the family is important when a child is born pre-maturely or has congenital problems. Specific needs require attention and teaching the new mother and the family how to care for twins, is important for long-term outcomes. Children's Medical Services (CMS) can provide financial help for care and teaching time for new mothers. The case manager coordinates CMS benefits with the patients' health insurance, to maximize available insurance benefits.

Pediatric Care Plan Goals

Case managers who specialize in pediatrics need to ensure that the care provided to children is illness- and patient-specific. Depending on the child's age, care is tailored to meet the normal growth and development of the child. The case manager ensures that the appropriate and least restrictive settings are used to provide care.

To understand the dynamic, complex growth and development of children, case managers review pediatric theorists to help them to address symptom management and compliance issues. Theorists provide insight about stages of growth and development by age group. For example:

- Piaget was a cognitive theorist who addressed children's abilities by age group, eg, the ability to synthesize and analyze information at the age of adolescence. Piaget can help case managers understand why reasoning with young children as to the need for a procedure will not be possible. Instead, encouraging parents and caregivers to support and comfort them during and after procedures are more effective. For example, when educating the mother of a five-year-old with cystic fibrosis about performing chest compressions, the case manager would not inform the mother to give the child a choice of when to do the therapy. Instead, comforting the child and spending time doing something he/she likes after therapy is a better way to approach a child's expected resistance.
- Erickson is a theorist who focused on children's social environment. His work helps case managers to understand peer pressures felt by children, which may make them noncompliant with medication or treatment regimes. An example that illustrates this theory is when a newly diagnosed diabetic teenager who wants to "fit in" does not follow his diabetic diet, resulting in consistently high blood glucose levels. The case manager who understands and acknowledges peer pressure can consult with a nutritionist to provide a diet that allows some flexibility when he is out with friends. By doing this, the case manager provides a way for the teen to "fit in" without compromising his health.
- Skinner is a theorist focusing on behavior. His research with monkeys proved the effectiveness of a reward system for appropriate behavior. Bargaining is an effective tool that works when dealing with school age children who are rewarded with special favors or favorite television shows when complying with treatments. Children with chronic illness sometimes feel less important than their peers. Rewarding them for taking their medication or doing their exercises daily is a way to boost self-esteem, and at the same time helping them learn how to manage their chronic illness.

Another challenge that health care professionals encounter is that of learning disorders or behavioral problems. Managed care case managers can provide referrals to specialists who are able to work with children who have learning disabilities and behavioral problems. Sometimes, cognitive or behavioral abnormalities can stem from an acute illness. Lead poisoning has been linked to behavioral and cognitive deficits in children. Attempts to remove lead from paint has been a goal in the U.S. for several years, but lead-based paint is still present in many older homes, especially in lower socioeconomic communities. Children who are hungry or bored sometimes eat paint chips peeled from walls. The effects of lead are slow to develop, but should be considered when behavioral or learning disorders are found. Also, women who are pregnant and consume fish that may be contaminated with chemicals or toxins, are at risk for toxins crossing the placental barrier, to enter the fetus. Studies show that infants and children exposed to toxins have alterations in behavior similar to those produced by lead.[13]

REFERENCES

1. Walthall, S. An enhancement of the role of clinical nurse specialist. *Michigan Nurse.* 2000: 63,5:6–8.
2, 3. Peplau, H. Is healthcare a right? *Image: Journal of Nursing Scholarship.* 1974: 7,1:4–10.
4. DuPen, A. Stanley, K. New directions in cancer pain management and assessment. Raritan, NJ; Ortho Biotech, Inc; 2000:4–5.
5. Llewellyn, A, Moreo, K. Essentials of case management: tools, techniques, principles and practices. Miramar, FL; Professional Resources In Management Education, Inc.; 2001:45–48.
6, 7, 11. Case Management Society of America. CMSA *Standards of Practice for Case Management Revised 2002.* Little Rock, AR. CMSA; 2002.

8. Mullahy, C. (1999). *The case manager's handbook.* 2nd ed. Gaithersburg, MD: Aspen Publication; 1998: 173–175.

9. Miles, J, Moreo, K. Dialogue and drilldown: achieving collaboration between case managers and physicians. *CMSA 10th Annual Case Management Conference Proceedings Manual.* Little Rock, AR; 2000: 216–226.

10. Moreo, K. Fatigue management in HIV/AIDS. *Advance for Providers of Post Acute Care.* 2000: 3,9:30–31.

12. Vohs, J.R. Family-centered case management: fundamental principles. *Surgeon General's Conference Proceedings Manual.* Washington, DC. US Government Printing Office; 1998.

13. Freidrich, M. Poor children subject to environmental injustice. JAMA. 2000: 283,5: 345–347.

REHABILITATION AND RETURN-TO-WORK 3

The first two chapters of this book present a view of the role and process of case management across multiple disciplines and through several health care settings. One setting is so unique and complex that it requires a personal tour—rehabilitation and its relationship in return-to-work. Historically, case managers have played a dynamic role in both rehabilitation of a patient and in returning an ill or injured person to gainful employment. Rehabilitation case management has been successfully practiced since the 1940s, when massive numbers of wounded soldiers returned from active duty in World War II. Case managers coordinated extended community services for soldiers requiring psychological healing long after their physical wounds healed.[1] While the role of the first rehabilitation case managers was different from the roles assumed by rehabilitation case managers in today's technologically advanced medical system, the needs of today's patients remain fundamentally the same as those of patients 60 years ago. These include:

- positive, ongoing adjustments to the dramatic changes occurring as a result of the illness or injury;
- improved quality of life;
- ongoing education and empowerment of the patient and family/caregiver regarding age-related and disability-related challenges and solutions;
- restoration or establishment of gainful employment.

Overall, the profile of patients requiring rehabilitation in today's environment is quite different from what it was even a decade ago. Rehabilitation programs today are seeing individuals with greater degrees of disability and longer life expectancies. Individuals are of all ages with diverse premorbid lifestyles, and variable support systems. They are entering the rehabilitation process earlier and are being sent home earlier at a level that is often less than completely independent, requiring more intense, creative discharge planning.[2] Further, the ongoing rehabilitation needs of injured or ill persons are becoming more complex, with more levels of recovery occurring in the home environment. Therefore, rehabilitation case management requires specific skills and services that include:

- ability to review and summarize medical records and progress reports;
- initial assessment of the patient that includes physical, behavioral, psychosocial, and financial evaluation of the patient, with added emphasis on family living arrangements, family dynamics, and any pre-morbid deficits that could affect community reentry and return to work;
- effective and ongoing collaboration with physicians and other health care providers to design an effective medical and vocational treatment plan;
- facilitation, coordination, and evaluation of necessary services;
- facilitation, coordination and evaluation of necessary supplies and equipment, including those that may not be a covered benefit, such as home and vehicle modifications;
- identification of quality, cost-effective alternatives for ongoing care, particularly in chronic and catastrophic cases;
- establishment of appropriate goals and timelines for the recovery process;

- communication with the patient's employer for potential return-to-work;
- facilitation of vocational and psychological counseling services;
- comprehensive reporting of ongoing clinical assessment;
- accounting of anticipated and actual medical and vocational expenses;
- community reintegration services;
- education and empowerment of the patient/family toward self-care.

The rehabilitation needs of patients dictates that these skills are used in a variety of circumstances, for a variety of reasons. Most of this chapter centers on the needs of the patient who can return to work as part of the rehabilitation process. This is because return-to-work is synonymous with rehabilitation in a large portion of the patient population. Many times, however, facilitating a patient's rehabilitation to maximum functional and psychosocial status will not entail a successful return-to-work. Successful rehabilitation of a child with cerebral palsy, for example, may indicate that the case manager's goal is to integrate the child back into the school system, coordinating the most appropriate level and intensity of schooling possible in the best interests of the child. Successful rehabilitation of the retired cancer patient may indicate that the case manager has empowered the patient to accept his/her disease and prognosis, and to begin lifestyle changes to enhance survival, such as improved meal planning, a moderate exercise program, and participation in a support group. Successful rehabilitation of the at-home mom may indicate that the case manager has mobilized community resources to assist the mother during her recovery period, including car pools, an affordable after-school care program, and delivery of prepared meals.

Regardless of the situation, the rehabilitation case manager is successful when a meaningful lifestyle has been achieved by the ill or injured patient. The skills sets presented earlier are applicable in all situations, and aid the case manager in moving the patient toward a meaningful lifestyle. Certainly, some of the skills and services delivered by rehabilitation case managers require more specialized training and expertise than others. The most profound of these skills sets involves vocational and return-to-work assistance. Time away from work affects both the employee and the employer. The employee loses all or a portion of his/her income, depending upon benefits offered by the employer. The employee also loses the social contact, sense of accomplishment, and day-to-day continuity gained from employment. The employer primarily experiences significant costs associated with work absence as lost productivity.

Consider the June, 2000 study of 11 telecommunications companies by the Integrated Benefits Institute. It demonstrated that the productivity lost when employees are away from work is a far greater financial burden to the company than the actual costs of benefits provided. The study confirmed that group health costs were 22%, disability and workers' compensation costs were 4%, and lost productivity was a disproportionate 74% of the companies' overall expenses.[3]

This certainly explains why vocational and return-to-work assistance by the case manager become very important skills sets in the rehabilitation process. This chapter addresses the many aspects of vocational and return-to-work processes that can be successfully performed or coordinated by the case manager. The first of these is job analysis.

JOB ANALYSIS

One process used by rehabilitation case managers in assessing a person's vocational needs is a job analysis. A job analysis objectively describes the job performed by the worker as well as defines the worker's functions and the physical requirements necessary to perform the job. It is a snapshot of what the worker does, how the work is performed, what are the expected worker characteristics, and what is the context of the work performed, including the environment, the organization, and the nature of responsibilities.[4]

In completing a job analysis, the rehabilitation case manager should perform an onsite assessment. He/she will gather information from the employer and from workers performing the same or similar functions as the job being analyzed. Personal observation and one-on-one interviews with peers and the employer remain key processes to obtain an accurate job analysis. When the rehabilitation case manager or specialist gathers this information, he/she can determine essential job functions for the stated job. Identification of essential job functions will assist the case manager to determine whether an injured/ill worker can perform the required tasks of the job. Identifying essential job functions is also a necessary component if the injured/ill worker wishes to establish his/her rights under the Americans with Disabilities Act (ADA). Information on the pertinence of essential job functions under the ADA is covered in Chapter eight of this book.

Essential job functions may also be identified in the injured/ill worker's job description. Accurate job descriptions are essential for each job in the workplace. The case manager will review the patient's job description to compare tasks that are indicated with what he/she actually observes during the onsite assessment. Accurate job descriptions are essential to provide the treating physician with appropriate information to determine the patient's ability to return to work.

When the rehabilitation case manager compiles data gathered into a job analysis report, the written report should include:

- Worker functions, which are those actions of the worker that relate to data, people, and things;
- What is achieved in the job;
- Identification of equipment, tools, and other work aids used to accomplish the tasks;
- Physical demands and work conditions;
- Environmental conditions;
- Worker characteristics required by the job, such as ability to deal with people, perform under stress, set limits and tolerance, and adapt to variety and change;
- MPSMS, which is an acronym that stands for materials, products, subject matter and services related to the job.

Because a job analysis is comprehensive, it should be performed only by rehabilitation professionals and case managers who have training in vocational evaluations. The results of a job analysis often define whether a need exists for job modification to return a disabled worker to gainful employment.

JOB MODIFICATION

An agreement by the employer to modify a job may happen for different reasons. In some cases, job modification occurs because the employee brings to the employer's attention compliance issues with the ADA (see Chapter eight), and the employer is required by federal law to modify certain aspects of the job description. In other cases, the worker may be a beneficiary of workers' compensation, and the case manager negotiates with the employer to modify certain job requirements to return the worker to gainful employment. This can occur if the worker's physician releases the employee to resume work duties, while defining clear limitations of work duties that are unsafe for the worker to perform. Employers are becoming more and more aware of the benefits of early return-to-work to obviate the costs of absenteeism and potential long-term disability claims.

There are also times when job modification results from a medical case manager advocating for his/her patient without having vocational experience. For example, an acute care case manager working in the hospital's outpatient chemotherapy unit could learn that a patient receiving chemotherapy treatment for his colon cancer is experiencing significant fatigue stemming from the treatment. The patient expresses fear to the case manager that he may lose his job due to his need to take frequent rest breaks during the day. He indicates that he must stop the chemotherapy treatments to keep his job and protect his family's finances. The case manager, with the patient's permission, contacts the patient's employer and explores how the worker's job might be modified. The employer agrees to allow the worker to modify his work schedule to half days, and to work from home one day a week. This is one example of job modification. Other forms of job modification may include limiting or eliminating certain physical tasks normally performed in the job, such as lifting or bending, or rewriting the job description to encompass other tasks able to be performed by the worker.

Employers play a critical and key role in job modification and in the overall success of an ill/injured employee's return-to-work. They are an integral part of what is known as the *three-point contact* by the case manager: communication with the patient, the primary physician, and the employer. It is extremely important for the case manager to communicate directly with the patient, the employer, and the physician, and to facilitate dialogue between the employer and the employee, as well as between the physician and the employee. This dialogue will help ensure that the employee can return to work in the same job capacity, or in an altered capacity within the same company. If this is not possible, the employer may be a valuable resource in suggesting or opening the door to suitable gainful employment available elsewhere.

The ultimate goal of the employer should be to maximize opportunities for the employee to return to suitable, gainful employment within the company, and to identify and initiate measures to enhance safety-in-the-workplace to prevent further similar injuries/accidents. The short-term goal of the employer should be to communicate and cooperate fully with the rehabilitation case manager, other members of the rehabilitation team, the employee and the insurer (if any) to maximize the quality and efficacy of the rehabilitation process.

JOB ACCOMMODATION

This chapter has explored how jobs can be modified to assist an injured or ill individual seek gainful employment. In addition to, or instead of, modifying the actual job, the job environment may require redesign to allow the ill or injured worker to adequately perform tasks. Changes to the actual environment are known as job accommodation. Job accommodations can also occur for a variety of reasons, ranging from federal compliance with the ADA, to voluntary assistance from an employer wishing to hire a valuable, disabled job applicant.

Job accommodations in the workplace can be far reaching or simplistic. A simple example of job accommodation is moving files from an upper file cabinet to a lower cabinet to accommodate a worker who has an impaired reach. More extensive accommodations would be necessary for a wheelchair-bound worker. These might include raising the desk and/or workstation for roll-under access; widening hallways and doorways to provide clearance for the wheelchair; and providing a handicap-accessible stall in the common rest rooms. It is important to note that under the ADA, job accommodations must be made in both the immediate work area, and in all common work areas to provide accessibility. Common work areas include lunchrooms, vending machine areas, lockers and rest rooms, lounges, and any other area accessed by workers. If a company sponsors a recreational sport and provides transportation to the event, the vehicle transporting the employees must also be accessible. Job accommodation is often addressed by ergonomists who are experts in the field of accessible design. Ergonomists and ergonomics are discussed later in this chapter. Barrier-free design factors are discussed in this chapter.

Many employers proactively make job accommodations to prevent further injuries in the workplace. These job accommodations are often directed by the company's occupational health nurse, who may also perform many case management functions on behalf of employees and families. The occupational health nurse may bring to the attention of the employer common problems in the work environment that can be adjusted to avoid or lessen injuries. Computer screens placed at an appropriate height can lessen neck injuries and back pain. Keyboards placed at the appropriate height can prevent carpal tunnel syndrome. These are examples of the wellness focus taken by occupational health nurses who understand the benefits of job accommodation.

WORK ADJUSTMENT AND WORK TRANSITION

Obviously, adjusting to a significant illness or injury can be very difficult for anyone. Fear, anxiety, anger, self-doubt, and confusion are just a few of the overwhelming emotions experienced by the injured or ill person. Health care professionals are educated to address these emotions and to encourage the patient to achieve as much confidence and empowerment as is possible in the wake of life-changing circumstances. However, most health care professionals are not prepared to deal with the vocational challenges faced by ill and injured persons returning to work or seeking transition to work. In these cases, a rehabilitation case manager, usually in collaboration with a vocational specialist, can assist both the patient and the health care team.

A transition to the work environment will be uneventful for some patients, and truly monumental for others. The rehabilitation case manager will want to engage the employer, co-workers, and the support of the patient's physician whenever possible to assist the patient in a transition to work. Initially, it will be important for the case manager to speak with the patient to learn the patient's perspective of his/her expectations, limitations, and abilities surrounding a transition to work. If the case manager is involved by referral to the case, he/she will need to contact the payer to clarify expectations, discuss benefits or coverage issues, and to determine other individuals involved in the care plan who should be contacted.

Upon meeting with or speaking with the patient to assess work adjustment and work transition needs, the case manager will want to explore the patient's expectations to return to work with the same employer or at another job. Vocational strengths of the patient should also be discussed, including whether the patient has any transferable skills that can be utilized working for another employer, or in a modified job for the same employer. This will require that the case manager understands the patient's past work history. The case manager will need to obtain permission from the patient to contact other essential individuals in the job transition process, including the patient's physician and the patient's employer.

Sample Template of Topics to be Addressed with the Patient

In order to adequately assess the patient's needs for work adjustment and work transition, the case manager should explore the following topics with the patient.

- Is the patient currently working? If not, when did he/she stop working?
- What is the patient's primary spoken language? Is the patient bilingual?
- Can the patient read and write? In what language(s)?
- Current medical status;
- Health status expectations and perceptions by the patient;
- Past medical history that could impact employability;
- Allergies;
- Medications the patient is currently taking;
- Noted barriers to work adjustment, such as amputation, paralysis, limp, unsteady gait, fatigue, dizziness, etc;
- Is the patient currently able to perform ADLs independently, or does he/she need help? If so, who is currently assisting and in what manner?
- Is the patient married? Living with someone? Who is the primary caregiver?
- Number of years of school completed;
- Any military experience.

By conducting a thorough and objective assessment of the patient's current status, including situational analysis and functional assessment, the case manager obtains valuable information, which will allow him/her to assess barriers and strengths in work adjustment or work transition. The case manager will gather information to allow insight into how the patient perceives and understands his/her current condition and the treatment plan that is in place. The case manager may also be able to gain insight into family dynamics. The past medical history is also explored in order to see how the current injury/illness may be affected by other conditions the patient may have. It is important to assess the patient's ability to speak and read English, as well as the number of years of completed schooling in order to gain insight into vocational issues that may arise in addition to the medical complications already facing the patient in work transition. All of these factors are important in developing a work adjustment/transition plan. As the case manager determines an effective transition plan for the patient, he/she must obtain approval of the plan from the patient.

Once the case manager has completed an interview with the patient, he/she will need to determine safety parameters involving transition to work. The patient must perform only those aspects of a job that are not a direct safety threat to himself/herself and others. The patient's physician should be contacted and provided with a written job description, provided by the employer, that defines the physical job demands, including the environment, physical and cognitive tasks, time requirements, and other pertinent data. Provided with accurate and appropriate job information, the physician can best determine whether the patient should have limitations to current job demands. The case manager should also provide a copy of his/her work transition plan to the physician, or discuss the plan with the physician if no formal written plan has been developed. A comprehensive plan will include short-term and long-term goals, as well as time frames in which the goals can be achieved. The goals must be specific, measurable, attainable, and relevant. Time lines are set up with each goal in order to make sure that the plan is re-evaluated.

After collaborating with the physician, the case manager should contact the employer to discuss the patient's abilities and limitations in a transition to work. Perhaps the limitations will be so severe that there is no return-to-work potential. Perhaps transition to work can be successfully achieved if the case manager can initiate efforts to provide job modification or job accommodation through the patient's existing employer. If return-to-work with the same employer is unlikely, perhaps the case manager will need to explore options for the patient to seek new employment.

VOCATIONAL ASPECTS OF CHRONIC ILLNESS AND DISABILITY

While a focus on rehabilitation and return-to-work strategies is required by legislation through workers' compensation systems across all fifty states, this focus has grown only as our understanding of the complex physical, emotional, financial, and behavioral issues surrounding profound illness and injury have matured. Providing rehabilitation and such services as job analysis, job modification, job accommodation, and work adjustment/transition is still not a responsibility of most health payer systems. Further, although these services are nationally covered in workers' compensation system, rehabilitation and vocational assistance have not always been addressed for workplace injuries.

CASE STUDY

Consider the documented case of an amputee injured on the job on May 8, 1930, at a cinder block company in St. Louis, MO. The 23-year-old male employee was cleaning a conveyor when he fell into the machinery, severing his right arm above the brachial region, receiving a compound fracture of the left leg, incurring extensive rupturing of the muscles and nerves of the left leg, damage to the right leg, and experiencing extensive tearing of the perineum and rectum. Subsequent to the accident, the injured worker sustained amputation of the right arm, permanent loss of the use of the left leg distal to the knee, lacerations and temporary muscle damage to the right lumbar region of the back and the abdomen, atrophy distal to the left leg injury, and permanent, partial loss of bowel function.

The injured worker spent one month in the hospital, and was discharged to home with follow-up care to be provided by his wife. He subsequently developed agitated nervousness and feelings of helplessness and hopelessness. Since there was no rehabilitation provided to this worker as part of the treatment plan, the injured worker's physician recommended the following in a written statement dated April 3, 1931: "I believe this man has now reached the point where he should make an effort to rehabilitate himself."

The Missouri State Workers' Compensation Commission determined the injured worker's status to be PPD (permanent partial disability) on September 30, 1931, and awarded him the maximum allowable payment for PPD—66 2/3% of his average weekly wage of $23.07 for 400 weeks, in a lump sum settlement of $6,152. Upon appeal of the case by the injured worker, the workers' compensation court ruled in denial of additional funding or any ongoing medical care, stating that the employee was subsequently engaged in gainful employment—he was peddling eggs, limping door-to-door in his neighborhood.

Consider this case by today's rehabilitation standards of care in a workers' compensation system. This same injured worker would have been immediately assigned to a catastrophic case manager, who would have coordinated a comprehensive rehabilitation team that likely would have included an orthopedic surgeon, a vascular surgeon, a general surgeon specializing in bowel function, a gastro-enterologist, a physiatrist, a pain specialist, a psychologist, a rehabilitation nurse, a physical therapist, an occupational therapist, a dietician, a social worker, and a vocational counselor. Following an acute care stay, the injured worker would have been transferred to a comprehensive inpatient rehabilitation facility for ongoing aggressive intervention by a similar specialized health care team. Weekly staffings by key members of the health care team would be used to report the injured worker's medical, psychological, and social progress toward short-term community re-integration. The injured worker and his wife would be actively involved in his ongoing care, with continual training, education, and support toward life-long adjustment and acceptance of the various deficits experienced.

Following successful inpatient rehabilitation, the injured worker would be transferred to home. The case manager would coordinate home health care services, using an agency specializing in catastrophic nursing and supportive care. The case manager would also coordinate wound care to include specialists in orthotics and prosthetics, durable medical equipment including disposables and incontinence products, assistive devices, compression therapy, bed support surfaces, ambulation aids, adaptive driving equipment and training services, home modifications and barrier-free architectural design. Care would also include life-care planning to address the lifelong needs of the injured worker, and to determine a fair settlement. A comprehensive vocational evaluation, would include job analysis, job modifications and accommodations, work hardening, and transitional counseling. If a new job was required, the worker would have vocational training, job development, and job placement to enable the injured person to begin a new career.

Clearly, return-to-work was not a focus in the Missouri workers' compensation system in 1930. Yet, today's rehabilitation case manager must have a broad knowledge base and skills regarding vocational aspects of disabled and chronically ill patients. The nature and scope by which a rehabilitation case manager can assist a patient in return-to-work will largely depend upon the payer system. The case manager must recognize which systems provide limited or no financial support for return-to-work, such as managed care health plans. In this scenario, the case manager will want to explore whether the chronically ill or injured patient qualifies for vocational services and wage loss benefits under other systems, such as vocational rehabilitation and Social Security Disability Income (SSDI). More information on these systems is provided in Chapter nine.

Rehabilitation case managers assisting a patient in return-to-work should engage the following sequential steps in determining how the person might return to gainful employment:

1. Modifications of the current job with the same employer, including a transitional return to work plan;
2. Exploration of a new job with the same employer, consistent with the patient's identified limitations and restrictions, and including work hardening, if necessary;
3. Modifications of a previous job with a new employer;
4. A new job with a new employer as a result of job placement, based on transferable skills and aptitudes;
5. A new job with a new employer involving on-the-job training;
6. A formal retraining and job placement.

Each of these sequential steps is covered in other sections within this chapter, as part of the overall vocational evaluation process. A vocational evaluation is a comprehensive process that systematically uses work, either real or simulated, as the focal point for assessment and vocational exploration. It incorporates medical, psychological, social, vocational, educational, cultural, and economic data gathered by the rehabilitation case manager or by a vocational specialist to determine goals and objectives in a vocational plan of care.[5] A vocational evaluation is used to:

- determine employability;
- identify barriers to return-to-work;
- identify services/products to overcome those barriers.

A properly performed vocational evaluation produces a vocational diagnosis for the patient, which includes the preparation of the person regarding both job readiness and employability of the person being evaluated. In cases where patients are severely disabled, such as with a traumatic brain injury, the employability of the person may be limited to very simple tasks. Still, if employability is possible, the evaluation has been successful. The employability of the individual becomes less focused on assisting the individual to earn an income, and more on lifelong rehabilitation. Employment of the person may be possible only through community resources, where the person works for a stipend, and is monitored closely and allowed to perform rehabilitation-enhancing tasks. The individual gains improved quality of life, and is able to be financially independent. Employment of the person may give the person's family some respite from the burden of caregiving. This example demonstrates the fact that a rehabilitation case manager is most successful when the person achieves a meaningful lifestyle.

WORK HARDENING RESOURCES AND STRATEGIES

Whether a disabled worker is adjusting to a modified job or seeking new employment because of limitations, it is imperative for the individual to learn new techniques that prevent re-injury and promote safety for both the worker and co-workers. Work hardening is a method, used to re-train a worker in physical techniques.

Work hardening, a specific rehabilitation program, uses a controlled, artificial environment similar to the injured person's actual work environment. This simulated environment may be at the company where the person will be assuming his/her former job, a modified version of his/her job, a new job; or, may be the perceived environment of a potential employer. The purpose of the artificial environment is to mirror, as closely as possible, the worker's actual job functions within the actual environment.

Before entering a work hardening program, the person participates in a functional capacity evaluation (FCE), usually performed by a physical therapist. The FCE allows the therapist to explore the person's ability to perform normal activities related to his/her job function, such as stooping, bending, lifting, etc. The results of the FCE enables the rehabilitation team performing the work hardening to develop a program suited to the person.

The work-hardening program is the final stage of physical therapy to prepare the person for return-to-work. A well-planned work hardening program enables the injured worker to safety and deliberately prepare for reentry into the work force. The work-hardening team may comprise a physiatrist, physical therapist, occupational therapist, nurse, pain specialist, vocational consultant, and an ergonomist. The team teaches such functions as proper lifting, squatting, bending, standing, positioning, and other body mechanics to maximize function and minimize risk of injury.

ERGONOMICS

Ergonomics is the process of adapting the work environment to meet the wellness needs of the injured or ill person. An ergonomist assesses the job environment to determine whether certain components can be modified or eliminated by redesign to prevent further illness or injury, and to promote wellness. As part of the environmental assessment, ergonomists address situations and conditions that may alter a person's optimal level of function. These include lighting, noise, workstation design, and distractions in the immediate area or the common areas of the work setting.

An example of ergonomic assessment for a chronically ill person focuses on a worker with chronic asthma. The worker's asthma is known to be triggered by extrinsic allergens, such as dust mites. An ergonomist examines the work area and determines that, in addition to keeping the worker's immediate workstation as clean and dust-free as possible, the common air conditioning system must be adapted to include an allergy-prevention filtration system. An example of ergonomic assessment for a worker with behavioral deficit focuses on the worker with diagnosed attention deficit disorder (ADD). Since the worker is easily distracted, the ergonomist determines that the employee's workstation must be removed from the existing cluster grouping, and placed in a private office with a door.

Ergonomic assessments can be done in a proactive manner to prevent injures from occurring on the job, and to promote wellness in the workplace. Over the past few years, ergonomics, as it relates to injury prevention, has focused primarily on the reduction of cumulative trauma disorders (CTDs).[6] CTDs are among the leading cause of workplace injuries, and include a wide variety of diagnoses such as tendonitis, bursitis, carpal tunnel syndrome, and several types of back problems. These syndromes result from overuse of specific muscles, tendons, ligaments, and joints and usually develop gradually over time.

Ergonomists are often asked to prevent or thwart an increase in CTDs. Risk factors for CTDs are position, force, and repetition. An example of CTD caused by position is the typist who types with her wrists bent, rather than typing with the wrists in a neutral position. The ergonomist evaluates risk factors for CTD in the work environment and makes modifications, such as placing a "lift" beneath a computer keyboard, making the employee's work easier to perform.

Ergonomists also assess products that enable workers to use near-normal postures that lessen force or repetition.[7] Examples include adjustable chairs, back /abdomen lift braces, knee pads, hydraulic-lift tables, anti-fatigue floor mats, workstation height extenders, and wrist rests. These products prevent injuries and decrease stress on vulnerable or healed areas.

VOCATIONAL ASSESSMENT

A vocational assessment is a comprehensive process conducted over a period of time to identify individual characteristics, skills, education, job training, and job placement needs of an ill or injured worker. The assessment usually involves a multidisciplinary team that plans an individual's educational program.[8] The role of the vocational specialist who assesses the worker and the work environment is to provide or enhance employment opportunities for the ill or injured worker. The vocational specialist may be completing a job search on behalf of the ill or injured worker, to maximize the person's ability to return to work, or to seek work once the rehabilitation process is complete. The vocational specialist may also evaluate the ill or injured person to determine his/her employability.

Vocational specialists have specific education to perform vocational testing and should be used as needed. The rehabilitation case manager must understand the scope of practice, and the practice within that setting. If the rehabilitation case manager is not prepared in vocational activities, he/she should refer the patient to a vocational specialist in a timely, efficient manner.

The vocational specialist and the rehabilitation case manager should function within the limits of their defined roles, education, and professional competencies, and should not recommend or request specific medical examinations, procedures, tests, or psychometric evaluations that are outside the scope of their education. Because few other health care providers focus exclusively on returning an ill or injured patient to work, the vocational specialist and the rehabilitation case manager together fill a critical role in maximizing vocational opportunities for an ill or injured patient seeking employment or return to work.

The vocational specialist uses different tools and tests as part of a vocational assessment. These include:

- Achievement tests (eg, reading comprehension tests)
- Aptitude tests (eg, motor coordination tests)
- Vocational tests (eg, ability to make correct choices to supervise others)
- Work samples (eg, testing both the ability to weld and the knowledge of welding)
- Behavioral observation (eg, patient's ability to follow directions during test-taking)
- Situational assessment (eg, observing patient's behavior in a simulated or role-playing work setting)
- Work trials (eg, observing the patient in the actual work setting)

Another common tool of the vocational specialist is a transferable skills analysis. Skills analysis is appropriate when the person's actual or projected physical abilities are too limited to allow the person to perform essential functions of the job. The ill or injured person is interviewed for past work history, education, and training. An analysis is then conducted to profile the past jobs, determining the highest level of vocational functioning. These functions are classified as transferable skills, because they are skills that the individual can use, or transfer, from one given job to another. An example of some of the transferable skills of a successful case manager include concise written and verbal communication skills, critical thinking, collaboration, and negotiation. Transferable skills are based on the individual's aptitudes, skills and physical abilities, and are documented to assist in determining current and projected employability of ill or injured persons.

A vocational specialist uses a labor-market survey as part of the vocational assessment/evaluation. A labor-market survey or analysis is often performed when an ill or injured worker requires retraining. The survey searches the local job market to determine job availability of jobs suited to the person's skills, abilities, and physical limitations. The survey, combined with information from the skills analysis, is used for:

- a job search;
- career counseling;
- the study of employment trends;
- a wage-loss analysis.

The steps a vocational specialist takes in completing a labor-market survey include determining the focus of the study, identifying the data-gathering method, and determining the final form of the data. In the past decade, Internet access has changed data-gathering methods. Vocational specialists are able to perform quick, efficient job searches. Major newspapers have online versions of their classified ads. Many employment entrepreneurs have websites as a way to capitalize on advertising opportunities generated by frequent site visitors ("hits"). Vocational specialists are advised to use good judgment to access both traditional and Internet-based sources when doing job searches.[9]

JOB DEVELOPMENT AND PLACEMENT

If the labor-market survey is done for career counseling, the vocational specialist is engaged in job development and placement for the ill or injured patient. Job development involves training or retraining a person for a new job or career change when the person cannot return to his/her pre-injury job, and no new position can be obtained based upon the individual's current transferable skills and physical limitations.

For example, a truck driver sustaining a low back injury in a weekend recreational activity cannot return to his job, which requires him to sit for long hours, exacerbating his chronic pain. The orthopedic physician treating the truck driver advises the patient to look for a more sedentary job, and suggests an office job where he may be able to take frequent stand-up breaks. With the help of the case manager at the hospital where he was initially treated, the truck driver identifies an independent vocational specialist, who completes a vocational assessment, documenting that the truck driver requires vocational training. The specialist refers the injured truck driver to vocational training services under the state's vocational rehabilitation program.

Once the truck driver successfully completes retraining in basic office and clerical skills, he is ready for job placement, and begins a search of the labor market, much as a vocational specialist conducts a labor-market survey. The difference is that a vocational specialist may conduct a labor-market survey for employability, whereas the truck driver is seeking place-ability. Place-ability and employability are very different. Place-ability is the chance a person has of gaining employment due to his/her job readiness, while employability is the capacity a person has to gain employment. A person may not be place-able because his or her job readiness is deficient. If the same truck driver fears a career change and does not believe he is capable of performing an office job, despite his retraining, he is not job ready. Therefore, his employability is strong, while his place-ability is weak. Vocational specialists will first assess an ill or injured person's job readiness in the event the person has successfully completed re-training but fails to follow through with potential job leads provided by the specialist.

BARRIER FREE ARCHITECTURAL DESIGN

Often the ability of an ill or injured person to seek employment has as much to do with architectural barriers as with vocational barriers. If an ill or injured person cannot be independent in his/her ADLs in the home environment, or cannot access the workplace in his/her wheelchair, it won't matter how much training or retraining the person has accomplished. Dependence, rather than independence, will keep the worker from working.

Barrier-free architectural design is so important to a disabled person's home and work environments that state vocational rehabilitation systems and workers' compensation systems provide benefits to pay for barrier-free environments. Barrier-free architectural design encompasses a wide variety of processes and identifiers, including universal design, home modifications, workplace retrofitting, and medical remodeling. The intent of barrier-free architectural design is to maximize a disabled person's independence, and provide an environment that is equally accessed by persons of all ages and all levels of abilities.

Barrier-free workplace and home environments are created by environmental access specialists. An environmental access specialist is classified with ancillary professionals as part of the health care team. Environmental access specialists typically build their practice and their expertise on their related professional licenses/certifications. Practitioners credentialed in environmental access include OTs, rehabilitation nurses, building contractors, engineers, and architects. The existing national certificate for an environmental access specialist is a CEAC—and is based on the specialist's related professional license/certification. The goal of the environmental access specialist is to provide a safe, cost-effective, and quality-designed home or workplace environment for the disabled person that will also maximize the person's independence and autonomy.

LIFE-CARE PLANNERS

Life-care planning is a comprehensive written document that acts as a care map to estimate the required medical, financial, psychological, spiritual, and social needs that a catastrophically or chronically ill/injured person requires over the lifespan. The professional who completes a life-care plan is known as a life-care planner, with specialty training, expertise, and practice in this rapidly growing and dynamic field. Many case managers are experienced life-care planners. Practitioners credentialed in life-care planning include nurse case managers, social workers, economists, vocational counselors, and rehabilitation counselors.

The intended recipients of a life-care plan are those with catastrophic injuries or those who have chronic, disabling conditions such as traumatic brain injury, spinal cord injury, amputation, multiple fractures, severe burns, premature birth, congenital anomalies, cancer, AIDS, and cardiopulmonary disease. A life-care planner conducts a comprehensive review of the ill or injured person's medical records, and reviews the person's work or school records. Patient and family interviews are conducted, including all members of the health care team. The life-care planner then investigates cost and availability of necessary services, equipment, and other resources required now, and those anticipated to be required for the rest of his/her lifetime. Diagnosis and prognosis are carefully documented to determine all expected complications, comorbid conditions, challenges, and quality of life issues affecting the individual now and, likely, in the future because of the illness/injury, including considering the medical, financial, social, behavioral, and cognitive aspects of the person's illness or injury. The final written report is comprehensive and compiled in a format that is understood by the patient, the family, the treatment team, the payer, and the legal system.

Life-care planners use a number of reliable tools to prepare a comprehensive life-care plan, including the U.S. Life Tables, to determine the life expectancy of a disabled individual, Present and Future Value Tables to project the value of today's dollar in the future health care and socio-economic climate, statistical data reports by economists, clinical guidelines, reports of experts in the field, significant research and literature reviews, and the life-care planner's own advanced practice and expertise to determine the future needs of the injured person.

Life-care planners can be identified and referred by claims representatives, defense attorneys, plaintiff attorneys, guardians, case managers, and others who may require a systematic way to determine projected services, products, and costs associated with a disabled person's survival and quality of life, both in the present and the future. The overall goal of the life-care planner is to define in a clear, accurate, concise, and unbiased manner the needs of the ill or injured person over his/her anticipated lifetime. The life-care planner must remain objective throughout, while preparing the life-care plan, regardless of the payer source requesting the plan.

REFERENCES

1. Riddick, S.N. Life care plan. In R.S. Howe (Ed.), *Case Management for Healthcare Professionals*. Chicago, IL. Precept Press, Inc; 1994: 189–193.
2. Hrodey, C.J. Neurorehabilitation: Working toward an independent and productive lifestyle. *Case Review*. 1997: 12,3:49–52.
3. Geddes Lipold, A. Managing the guy who isn't there. *Business and Health*. 2000: 11,25:25–30.
4, 5, 8. Moreo, K. *Disability management and rehabilitation specialist handbook.* Miramar, FL: Professional Resources In Management Education Inc. Miramar, FL; 2000: 25–30.
6, 7. Melnik, M.S. Practical ergonomics: Inviting participation in an ergonomics process. *Case Review*. 1997; 12,3:55–58.
9. Kuhn, P, Skuterud, M. Job search methods: Internet versus traditional. *Monthly Labor Review*. U.S. Bureau of Labor Statistics. Washington, D.C. U.S. Government Printing Office. 2000.

DATA MANAGEMENT

4

Pressures from payers, providers, government officials, accreditation bodies, and the public continue to demand that the health care system find ways to contain escalating health care costs while, at the same time, to provide quality, accessible care. Critical to meeting this demand are information technology (IT) systems that are effective, efficient, and have a universal design—a common platform that allows a system used in one sector, such as the payer sector, to "talk" to the system in another sector, such as an integrated delivery system.[1]

Providers and payers across the country are searching for the right system to meet their diverse needs. They are purchasing new systems or making upgrades to existing systems in order to keep pace with the industry. To compete in today's dynamic health care environment, payers and providers must have IT systems able to sort through a vast amount of data to extract pertinent, objective information that supports the work they are doing in terms of quality, cost, and access. Information technology allows payers and providers to reduce errors by improving documentation and enhancing communication. Good IT systems use existing data to report outcomes, improve quality by objectively evaluating practice, and analyze and justify costs associated with a myriad of services delivered.

Because of the tremendous number of technical changes that have occurred in the last decade, keeping pace with these advances has challenged health care professionals to develop new technical skills and use tools that enable care to be streamlined. From an administrative standpoint, providers and payers are incorporating systems that allow information to be shared across the continuum of care. This integration has led to a decrease in variation in practice, and a reduction in the vast amount of administrative paperwork that results in fragmentation of care and increased costs.

Their role in controlling costs requires case mangers to have an understanding of the financial implications associated with health care. An integrated data management system allows case management professionals to demonstrate clinical, financial, and quality outcomes. Case managers have the opportunity to use their clinical knowledge and expertise by joining professionals called upon to design data management systems. By contributing to this process, the case manager ensures that systems are designed to meet the needs of the end user, while delivering outcomes to support and improve the practice. This chapter will give the case manager guidelines and information to achieve this goal, which can promote effectiveness and efficiency in providing services.

INDIVIDUAL AND AGGREGATE DATA COLLECTION

Traditionally, case managers have focused their attention on meeting the needs of the individual patient. With advances in information technology over the past few years, payers and providers are able to collect detailed data that expands the focus on outcomes to meet the complex health needs of the entire population. Armed with information, payers and providers are able to critically look at the population they are responsible to manage, and develop individualized programs to enhance wellness, while effectively addressing chronic illness and disease. This is accomplished by collecting data that allow stratification of the population according to specific disease processes. Stratification provides a clearer picture of how the population is managing their specific disease processes. This information gives users

59

the ability to stratify members according to risk, and develop a plan to proactively address potential problems. Data compiled from the aggregate population also provide critical information of what the cost of care will be to manage this population. This information is clearly valuable for both the payer and provider when contracts to provide care are negotiated.

When considering how IT affects case management, remember that the overall principle guiding the practice of case management is early identification of patients who are at risk for complications. Risk stratification allows this principle to be put into practice. Individual patients from the aggregate population can be triaged into case management early, so that problems can be addressed in a proactive manner, rather than retroactively. Disease management programs that focus on a particular disease use this concept to provide consistency and coordination to the process of care delivery.[2]

A patient with renal disease is an excellent example to illustrate this principle. Management of the patient with renal disease poses significant challenges because of the variety of health problems that can accompany this disease. Proactive management of comorbid conditions, including diabetes, hypertension, anemia, congestive heart failure, nutritional deficiencies, and atherosclerosis improves the quality of life of the patient and can lengthen the time before the patient will require permanent dialysis. Case managers from the payer or provider side who are called to individually manage a renal patient need to monitor data such as lab values, weight, and vital signs, while analyzing information gained from screening tools used to assess how the patient is managing his/her activities of daily living. The results gleaned from this information give the case manager important clues as to how the patient is doing, what specific problems are occurring, and how a plan of care can prevent an exacerbation. If these complex data can be collected, compiled, compared, analyzed, and accessible at the same time to all members of the health care team, continuity of care and consistency in care can be achieved. The patient's quality of life, functional status, and adherence to treatment can all be substantially improved through collaborative interventions. In retrospect, information from the patient's treatment and care plans can also be measured to evaluate the effectiveness of the overall process.

Collection

The perfect system to meet the needs of all users has yet to be developed. Ongoing research and development continue to improve systems that allow clinical and financial information to be collected, and the ability of systems to interface. For systems to be efficient and effective, it is important for organizations and individual departments to identify the information and data needed to perform their respective roles with maximum efficiency.

In the acute care setting, case managers care for patients during a single episode. However, information regarding any preceding episodes would be helpful as decisions are being made about the care required during the inpatient stay. For example, a 73-year-old man comes into the ED at 2:00 am from a local skilled care facility. He is confused and unable to provide any information. It is noted that he has left-sided weakness, a thready pulse, and blood pressure of 90/50. The initial impression is a CVA. Information regarding past history, medications taken, and the availability of advance directives would be very helpful to determine the possible cause of this event, and the ultimate treatment required to restore the patient's health and prevent future episodes. Similarly, information regarding the inpatient episode will be needed by other health care teams who will manage the patient as he continues to move through the continuum of care.

This example provides insight into how collection of data in one setting can allow a cohesive plan of care to be followed by subsequent providers. By collecting and building pertinent information from each episode of care, providers can gain a clear picture of each event that the patient has encountered. On an aggregate level, the data gathered provide information that can be analyzed and reported according to the needs of the provider or payer. For example, many payers develop and manage educational programs for their plan members in order to promote wellness and minimize illness/injury. Data regarding an increase in diagnostic testing, such as mammograms, could indicate to the payer that educational efforts are being effective and showing positive results. Data can be useful in identifying problems early, to improve prognosis, ability to treat problems, and obtain successful outcomes.

Likewise, the quality and effectiveness of decision-making depend on accurate, timely, and relevant information. To obtain accurate information, data must be entered accurately. Staff training is essential to ensure that each person understands the information that the data system provides to individual practice, and to the organization.

Security measures must be implemented to ensure that the integrity of the system is maintained. One way to ensure this is to require each person who has access to the system to have a password. Depending on the user, only certain areas may be able to be accessed to provide safeguards for patient confidentiality and security. Patient security within IT systems is promulgated through the federal Health Insurance Portability and Accountability Act (HIPAA). The intent is to protect the rights of the patient, while improving the efficiency and effectiveness of the health care system by standardizing electronic transmissions of patient information.[3] This legislation can have tremendous impact and implications for nearly every sector, if not every sector of the health care system. More information on this Act and on patient security is covered in Chapters eight and ten.

Application

Applications are tools used to integrate information to define standards of care, measure outcomes, examine variances, and make logical decisions and changes to the care process.[4] Each organization has different needs that require unique software applications. It is important to remember that it is not necessary to understand how each application works; rather, it is important that there is a clinical knowledge base to ensure that information reported is logical to the health care process. Knowledge is the fuel that allows software applications to work. Understanding the functions of an application will assist the user to maximize a given software program. Applications typically have three types of technical functions: presentation, business logic, and the database. Presentation controls how the application looks and feels. Business logic contains rules, edits, and logic for processing and input of data.[5] Commercial applications that are available are programs such as Excel™ and Access™. These programs allow information to be collected and incorporated into charts or databases to analyze and present information in an organized manner.

Several organizations prefer to customize their own programs rather than buy a ready-made system. Some organizations have an IT department that develops applications to meet the needs of the organization. If this is not available, an alternative is for the organization to contract with consultants who specialize in software development. Understanding and communicating what the needs are and what the organization wishes to accomplish is critically important to the overall success of the process. Accordingly, case managers must take an active role in defining and communicating their unique needs when applications or systems decisions are being made.

Analysis

The marketplace is demanding that health care providers and payers develop and provide data to improve care, support/define costs, and demonstrate outcomes. To do this, pertinent data generated every day by all involved in the health care system need to be analyzed. Computerized systems allow organizations to obtain information and generate reports on a variety of topics from the data collected. These include clinical information, logistical aggregate data, encounters with providers or payers, and financial information corresponding to services provided.

If a quality management team wants to evaluate the effectiveness of a particular treatment guideline or critical pathway, data generated from those using the pathway can be analyzed to determine variances in care and outcomes that may have occurred. Information gathered from analysis of these areas allows the team to determine whether the guideline or pathway is being used, applied effectively, and is meeting the desired goals. Data can also demonstrate whether changes in treatment patterns by physicians and ancillary professionals have occurred since the guideline or pathway was implemented. Important questions to be asked include:

- Has length of stay been reduced?
- Has variation in care been decreased?
- Are resources being used more appropriately?
- Can specific outcomes be captured in terms of cost, quality, and access to care?

Answers to these questions are part of the analysis of continuous quality improvement within an organization. Analysis, therefore, is a cornerstone of the IT system.

Evaluation

Information systems enable decision makers to choose a course of action that has the highest expectation of favorable results, both in terms of clinical and financial impact. Through a careful evaluation of the data, changes, procedures, and policies can be implemented so that systems can be improved. For example, the cardiac cauterization department may want to evaluate its efficiency and effectiveness compared to other cardiac cauterization programs in the region. Information that can be generated from the IT system can determine:

- the number of procedures performed within a given month/year;
- information concerning the type of patients selected for the procedure;
- outcomes of the procedure;
- the benefit/complication rate of the procedure;
- the cost of the procedure and the time to complete the procedure.

The results of this information can serve as a benchmark to show where the hospital stands in relation to other hospitals providing a similar service. Depending on the results obtained, action can be taken. If the outcomes of the information show that the cardiac cauterization program has excellent results using these variables, this information can be used to market the program to payers and the community. Conversely, if the outcomes demonstrate poor results, the data will be helpful to decide what changes need to be made to improve processes.

Reporting

Reports generated by an IT system should give the user adequate, objective information to review data critically. The data contained in the report should provide information that meets the stated goals of the analysis. Reports can include:

- clinical and/or financial data to support outcomes;
- activities (clinical and financial) that show service delivery to a specific population and whether the service was effective;
- objective information about overall services and care delivery within a specific population, and what outcomes were achieved.[6]

If changes are made as a result of the data collected, a follow-up report should be completed to evaluate the changes made, and to determine whether they were successful in correcting or improving the process. Organizations that establish efficient ways to collect and manage data will be able to obtain valid reports to measure success.

PROCESSES

The process of evaluating data to report outcomes begins with determining the goals that are to be achieved. As the emphasis on the delivery of quality, cost-effective patient care increases, comparing outcomes across settings becomes essential. To determine how an organization or provider performs when compared with similar organizations, it is to necessary to identify commonly used measures. This section will look at various tools of case management to measure processes.

Benchmarking

Benchmarking is an ongoing system of measuring products, services and practices against competitors or leaders in a given specialty. Benchmarking assists providers to improve their practice by measuring, evaluating, and comparing both results and processes that produce the best results. Benchmarking is part of the continuous quality improvement process used to improve processes by identifying those areas that need improvement. A facility that specializes in heart transplants may look at national standards to see how their particular program measures compared to other transplant centers. Length of stay, infection rates, and rejection rates are some indicators that are important to benchmark in this setting. If the facility ranks high in post-transplant infection, they will review their internal processes to make changes that will lower infection rates. After a certain time period, the facility then re-evaluates the data to determine whether changes occurred. This process of benchmarking allows organizations to remain competitive in terms of quality, cost effectiveness, and efficiency.

Best Practice Profiling

Best practice in the health care setting is viewed as a service, function, or process that has been fine-tuned, improved and implemented to produce superior outcomes. Providers strive to achieve best practices to ensure that the services and products they offer are of high quality and meet consumers', payers', regulatory and accreditation organizations' guidelines and expectations. Best practices result from benchmarks that allow organizations to meet or set new standards. Best practices are used to:

- improve clinical outcomes;
- improve administrative efficiencies;
- reduce costs;
- provide supportive data in growing market shares and contracting.[7]

Best practices are not unique to the health care industry. Businesses, academic institutions, and other organizations have been incorporating best practices into their structures for a number of years. Throughout the health care system, case management is one process being used to promote best practices in health care delivery. Effective case management improves the efficacy of care while promoting improved quality of care to gain patient satisfaction. Efforts by case management organizations to define and use best practices within the health care environment are an effective way to confront the changes and demands affecting health care organizations.

To define and use best practices within the health care environment, case mangers need to understand what consumers of health care want or expect. Much time and money are spent on process improvement, yet consumers' demands continue to be unmet. The Picker Foundation performed a study in 1997 that reflects the current dissatisfaction of consumers with health care. The study asked consumers what they wanted from the health care industry. The findings showed that most concerns could be grouped into eight dimensions of patient-centered care:

- the need to respect a patient's value preferences and expressed needs;
- the need to be able to access care;
- the need for emotional support;
- the need for information and education;
- the need for improved coordination of care;
- the need for physical comfort;
- the need for involvement of family and friends;
- the need for continuity and transition of care.[8]

To achieve best practices in the health care system, case managers and other health care professionals must listen to patients and families, and work to develop practices that meet stated demands. As advocates, case managers can lead this effort through collaboration with providers and payers. Incorporating best practices across the continuum of care will decrease fragmentation, maximize adherence, and improve quality of care, which will result in an overall reduction in health care costs and the assurance that precious resources reach those patients who have the greatest needs.

Cost-Benefit Analysis

Cost-benefit analysis is used to demonstrate the dollar-spent-to-savings- achieved ratio. In case management, documentation of savings achieved as a result of case management intervention, or as a result of implementation of a service or product, is an important outcome that the case manager can use to demonstrate his/her value to the health care system. Components that are included in the cost benefit analysis are:

- identifying information regarding the patient;
- overview of the case management intervention;
- summary of intervention;
- costs associated with case management intervention;
- any savings achieved. These can include:
  - Avoided charges
  - Potential charges
  - Discounts or negotiated rates
  - Reduction in equipment and services
  - Gross savings (potential minus actual charges)
  - Net savings (gross savings minus case management fees)
  - Status of case (open or closed).
- Review of pertinent aspects of the case including:
  - Clinical
  - Social-Situational
  - Educational
  - Wellness

The summary of the cost-benefit analysis should outline the case manager's specific intervention on the case. Issues included are the patient's compliance, enhancement of quality of care, outcomes achieved, prevention of greater illness or injury, and better/more appropriate use of resources.[9]

An example to illustrate this concept is when an independent case manager is called to work with a 68-year-old woman with peripheral vascular disease, who has had four acute care admissions in the past two months due to cellulitis. The managed care case manager assigned feels that an onsite case manager is needed to find out what factors may be causing the need for frequent admissions. Her supervisor authorizes the contracting of an independent case manager to perform a consultation.

After receiving the referral from the managed care case manager, the independent case manager calls the patient and makes an appointment to see the woman in her home. The patient is found at home, sitting on a recliner with her leg elevated. The case manager notices that the leg is swollen and has an old dressing, which is falling off, and is partially covering a large, oozing wound. The case manager discovers several things that may be contributing to the poor wound healing and exacerbation of the cellulitis. The case manager observes that the patient lives alone in a small, third-floor apartment. She is not able to drive to the store to get the prescribed supplies for her wound care. She states she has a few supplies from when she left the hospital, but she cannot remember how to use them as demonstrated by the nurse in the hospital. She states she does not want to bother her family since they are all very busy. The patient admits she is a heavy smoker, which could be contributing to poor circulation. The patient states she assured her doctor she would stop smoking, but she needs help.

Upon returning to her office, the case manager calls the treating physician to discuss the case. He states that he thinks the patient should be readmitted so that the social worker can find a skilled care facility for her to stay in until her wound heals. He does not know what to do for her anymore. The case manager recommends to the doctor that a course of outpatient physical therapy may be a solution. She states that in her review of the records, the patient's wounds began to heal each time she receives whirlpool therapy in the hospital. She suggests arranging for a series of outpatient whirlpool treatments. She also states that the therapy visits will allow professionals to clean and redress the wound, while increasing the woman's circulation stemming from activity. She assures the physician that she will keep him informed of progress and notify him if the wound is not healing effectively so that admission can be arranged.

The doctor agrees to the plan and states he will provide a script for whirlpool therapy three times a week with dressing changes. The case manager uses this opportunity to inform the physician that transportation is a problem, and that she anticipates the woman will be compliant with therapy only if she receives dependable third-party transportation, since it is highly unlikely she will contact her family for assistance. She also uses the opportunity to address the patient's smoking. She inquires whether the patient is a candidate for a nicotine patch to help her decrease the number of cigarettes she smokes. The doctor agrees to write a prescription for nicotine patches and third-party transportation for therapy.

The case manager calls the managed care case manager and informs her of the progress, gaining approval to proceed with coordination of the outpatient therapy. Expectedly, the nicotine patch and transportation are denied as uncovered benefits. Anticipating this denial, the independent case manager informs the managed care case manager that she has prepared a brief cost-benefit analysis, demonstrating the expected ongoing costs if the patient does not quit smoking and cannot get to therapy. The independent case manager informs the managed care case manager of the patient's history of refusing to seek assistance from her family, coupled with the other reasons for her repeated hospitalizations. She states that the third-party transportation and the nicotine patches are very small expenditures compared to even one additional hospitalization, which the physician is planning as an alternative treatment.

The managed care case manager is able to deliver the estimated cost-benefit analysis report to her company's medical director, who approves the out-of-benefit items. The independent case manager contacts an outpatient rehabilitation center in the managed care network and close to the woman's apartment that is equipped to provide the prescribed therapy. The case manager inquires about any wellness programs provided by the rehab center and learns that they provide smoking cessation classes. The case manager speaks with the physical therapist, who agrees to plan the therapy to coincide with these smoking cessation classes. The center also provides transportation for its patients.

The case manager speaks to the patient regarding her findings, and the patient is agreeable and thankful for the help. Therapy is scheduled to begin. The case manager follows the patient's progress over the next few weeks. In speaking with the physical therapist, she learns that the patient's wounds are showing signs of healing. The therapist informs her that the patient has been attending the smoking cessation classes, in addition to using the patch, and has been able to decrease from smoking two packs a day to less than a pack a week. The therapist states that she is going to recommend to the doctor in her report that the wound care treatments continue, but decrease to twice a week. The case manager speaks with the patient who states she is doing much better. She states this is the first month she is not in the hospital in a long time, and is very proud that she is able to cut down on her smoking. She is getting around the house more and should be able to start driving soon.

The treating physician is pleased that the patient is finally making progress. After another month all treatments are completed, the wound has healed, and the patient is back to her normal activities. The case manager speaks with the managed care case manager and suggests case closure. As part of her final report, the case manager includes a detailed cost-benefit analysis. The report demonstrates that, prior to case management involvement, the patient had four admissions, each lasting about five days. The average cost for each admission was $1,800/day, for a total of $36,000 in a short treatment period, excluding all intermittent physician visits. Care and costs implemented as a result of the case manager's intervention include outpatient physical therapy three days a week for three weeks, then two days a week for one month. The cost of therapy was $125 per treatment. The total cost for the outpatient therapy amounted to $2,125. There was no charge for the smoking cessation program or the transportation. The cost of the nicotine patches totaled $145. The independent case manager charged $75 an hour. She included 10 hours of intervention in the cost benefit analysis for a total of $750. To recap, the following charges were included in the cost-benefit analysis:

Expenses:
   Cost of physical therapy: $2,125
   Cost of nicotine patches $145
   Cost of case management services: $750
   Total Expenses: $3,020

Savings Achieved:
   Avoidance of additional 5 days of hospitalization: $9,000
   Direct Savings for the Case: $6,750

The savings in this report are known as "hard savings" because a dollar amount is depicted. There are also potential savings resulting from the case manager's interventions, such as reduced incidence of PVD exacerbations due to smoke cessation and increased mobility. These potential savings are known as "soft savings". Overall, the cost-benefit analysis report definitively demonstrates that, with case management intervention, the patient's clinical and functional status are improved, and quality of life is enhanced with avoidance of additional hospitalization. This example also illustrates how a cost-benefit analysis can be used at different times and for different reasons—in this case, two reports were used to achieve both out-of-benefit approval, and to demonstrate a hard savings outcome.

Many times, case managers impact or effect change with patients with whom they come in contact, but have difficulty demonstrating savings as a result of each intervention. Soft savings are often the result of education that the case manager may provide, or guidance that allows a patient to understand his or her disease process better, or to accept an aspect of the illness that was not previously understood. This understanding may result in the patient taking a more active role in his/her health care.

An example is a patient with hypertension. The ED case manager may take the time to talk to a patient who has come into the ED with headaches. In talking with her after she had been medicated for pain, the case manager finds that the patient had run out of her medication and did not have time to go to the clinic to obtain a new prescription. The case manager reviews with her the importance of taking her medications to prevent serious complications, such as renal disease or a stroke. By gaining a better understanding of the risks of noncompliance, the patient can see where her actions may lead, and vows to take better care of herself. Since these types of interactions occur continuously and fluidly in case management, case managers often don't take the time to document the teaching or the potential cost savings of their interventions. At the very least, documentation of the intervention is important. The result may be a behavioral change—a soft savings from improved self-care management. Improvement in quality of life is also a soft outcome that many times will have an impact on costs down the line, but in the short term may have a far greater impact for the person involved.

Peer Review

Peer review became the norm in 1975 when the Social Security Act created a nationwide review agency known as the Professional Standards Review Organization (PSRO). This organization was formed to ensure that medical care provided to patients was of high quality and reflected the most appropriate and efficient use of health care services.[10] Today, various accrediting bodies have replaced the efforts that the PSRO started. Organizations such as the Joint Commission on Accreditation of Healthcare Organizations (JCAHO), the National Committee for Quality Assurance (NCQA), and the American Accreditation Health Care Commission/URAC (URAC) are major organizations that provide quality, peer review oversight for health plans and health care organizations. These accreditation bodies require policies and procedures to be established to ensure that the care provided to patients meets high standards, and that health care professionals who provide care maintain competencies that can be measured and reported to the public.

Case management professionals play an important role in assisting their organizations and institutions to meet standards set by these organizations. Quality improvement programs ensure that the staff has the necessary credentials to perform services that are offered. Case managers may be involved in internal peer-review activities as part of their role. Peer review activities need to be handled confidentially due to sensitive information that can be discovered.

Peer review activities are meant to improve practice and not be punitive in nature. Many times, the medical director overseeing the case management department will communicate with another physician who has been over-utilizing diagnostic tests, according to information collected by the case managers. The medical director will discuss the information with the physician and may suggest ways that the physician can change and improve practice behaviors. Likewise, the acute care case manager may discuss a case with the nurse manager on a unit she covers regarding nursing behavior she feels may be impacting effective patient care. Case mangers have a responsibility to raise issues with the appropriate members of the health care team, since the case manager in the role of coordinator is often in the best position to objectively define peer problems.

Variance Tracking

Case management professionals use variance tracking as a way to reduce and/or manage negative occurrences related to the care provided to patients. Variance tracking can also identify positive occurrences that may then recognized as a standard of care to enhance practice. Variances can occur for several reasons. The following are some examples of negative variances:

- Patient variance: can occur when a complication arises from a procedure or treatment. An example of a patient variance is when a patient who is undergoing a closed MRI is unable to complete the procedure because of an anxiety attack. The delay in concluding the test causes an extended stay and a delay in the diagnosis.
- Clinician variance: is described as any untoward occurrence related to the clinician or professional charged with caring for a patient. An example of when a clinical variance would occur would be if the same patient were able to complete the MRI test, but there was not a radiologist available to read the MRI. This would result in a delay in diagnosis and potentiate an extended stay.
- System variance: A variance occurs when there is a breakdown related to the health care system in general. An example of a system variance would be when a neurologist orders an MRI for a patient admitted on a Friday afternoon, and is informed that the test cannot be performed until Monday, since the acute care hospital does not have a technician to perform MRIs over the weekend. The system is responsible for the variance that will cause an extended stay, and may likely be responsible for the cost of the unnecessary hospital days, since payers often deny payment resulting from delayed days in this type of variance.

Variance tracking allows an organization to identify areas where problems are occurring and critically evaluate whether changes need to be made. In the examples above, if the variance is impacting the safety of the patient or adversely impacting reimbursement, making change to correct the variance can be a recommendation by the case manager. Documentation regarding how the variance occurred, along with supporting information on associated costs, provides objective data that can be used to support the need for change. Further information on variance tracking is included under clinical guidelines in this chapter.

TOOLS

Case managers have many tools that enable them to evaluate how providers and other health care professionals within the health care system provide care to patients. For any tools to be used effectively, several things must be put into place. To have buy-in from those who will use these tools, it is important that the entire team involved in the treatment or procedure is also involved in developing the tool(s).

Education for those who will be involved in using the tools is also essential to ensure the tools are used for the intended purpose(s). Education should be done prior to implementation of the tool, and reinforced as part of the ongoing monitoring. It is important that the team understands that tools are not meant to replace clinical judgment, but are used to guide and organize treatment decisions in specific situations.

After the tools are developed, it is important to properly train staff about how to document the results generated from using the tools. For the tools to be viewed as a way to improve practice and not as a disciplinary measure, it is important that the tools are used to improve clinical practice and to decrease variation in care. This next section will address the various tools that are used in today's health care system.

Algorithms

Algorithms are systematic procedures that follow a logical progression based on additional information or a patient's response to an intervention to reach a solution for a specific problem. Like protocols, algorithms are a series of treatment steps, each of which is defined by the clinical response of the patient to the preceding step. However, unlike protocols, algorithms are research-based and have scientific support data. One of the most recognized uses of algorithms is in advanced cardiac life support. Professionals use a specific algorithm that relates to specific cardiac rhythms. Corresponding treatment is designed to interrupt an abnormal rhythm in an attempt to normalize the rhythm. The use of algorithms has helped to standardize emergency treatment, both inside the health care setting, and in the community, to provide treatment in an organized and efficient manner, to achieve successful outcomes.

Clinical Guidelines

Clinical guidelines are used in the health care industry to ensure that clinical interventions are less variable, are based on sound consistent practice, and optimize the management of limited resources. Clinical practice guidelines have emerged as a tool that health care professionals can use to improve the quality of care provided while controlling costs. Clinical guidelines are defined as systematically developed statements that assist the practitioner, health care team, and patients in making decisions about appropriate health care for specific clinical circumstances. Guidelines should be practice-based, patient-specific, and user-friendly. Key components that should be considered when developing clinical guidelines include:

- identification of key decisions and their consequence(s);
- review of the relevant, valid evidence on the benefit, risks, costs, and alternatives of each decision;
- presentation of the evidence regarding key decisions in a simple, accessible format that is flexible to the stakeholder's preference.[11]

Several organizations have developed websites that case managers, health care professionals, and the general public can access when they need information on clinical guidelines. Case managers can use these sites to gather information that will assist them to more fully understand a patient's diagnosis and treatment options. Clinical guidelines that incorporate practice-based or evidence-based medicine are important in today's health care environment. For a guideline to be considered evidence-based, it must go through rigorous study to ensure that scientific evidence demonstrates clinical effectiveness.

Two sites that offer excellent information are The National Guideline Clearinghouse™ (NGC) and the W.H. Kellogg Health Library. NGC is a public resource sponsored by the Agency for Healthcare Research and Quality (AHRQ) in partnership with the American Medical Association and the American Association of Health Plans. The website to access the Clearinghouse can be found at www.guideline.gov. Another resource, The W. H. Kellogg Library, is a site that contains guidelines based on evidence-based medicine. The website access to this information is located at www.library.dal.ca/kellogg.

Clinical Pathways

A clinical pathway is a tool that outlines all of the components of care for a patient with a particular diagnosis within a specific time frame. Pathways are ways of visualizing the process of care for a specific condition that a physician or nurse may encounter from day to day. Clinical pathways are also classified as critical pathways. Both are interdisciplinary in that they provide written criteria to guide the care delivery of multiple disciplines. Pathways delineate necessary treatment for a specified population of patients, facilitate appropriate resource use, and provide a standard for comparing actual with expected practice outcomes.

A clinical pathway is illustrated on a grid outlining the treatment on one axis, and the stated timeline with expected outcomes on the other axis. Categories that can be listed include such items as assessment and evaluation, diagnostic tests, consults, treatments, medications, diet, teaching, and discharge planning. An important element in the design of a pathway is the timeline. A timeline is a specified period over which an event is expected to occur. Timelines can vary according to where the path is used. In the emergency department, time may be measured in minutes or hours. In the acute care setting, where a diagnosis needs to be made, the length of stay can range from days to weeks. Usually, Diagnostic Related Groups (DRGs) are used as guides to determine length of stay. Months may be used to plot a course of treatment in areas such as the neonatal intensive care unit or a long-term care facility, where treatment is extended because of the nature of the problems and patients served.

For pathways to be accepted and used in clinical practice, a multidisciplinary approach is important to use when designing a clinical path. Health professionals who are involved in the treatment of patients, and who use the pathway should be included in all aspects of the pathway design, implementation, and evaluation. For example, in designing a myocardial pathway, the following professionals or departments should be included as the pathway is designed: cardiologist, nursing, respiratory therapy or a representative from the cardiopulmonary department, nutritionist, social services department, cardiac rehabilitation, and home health care. To prepare the staff who will incorporate the pathway into practice, an educational in-service should be held to introduce the path and explain to each department how the path is to be used, and documentation that accompanies the pathway.

The case manager can use this tool as a way to proactively identify problems, determine where the problems arose, and gather data that objectively provides information on how improvements to care or processes can be made. The case manager is able to objectively see how the patient is doing as a result of the use of clinical pathways, since the case manager has a broad view of the process. The case manager does this by continuously assessing whether the patient is meeting the expected goals of the pathway. If goals are not achieved, the case manager documents this as a variance.

Variances can occur at any time throughout the course of treatment. Variances occur when the patient does not progress as outlined according to the clinical pathway. Variances are usually classified according to who or what caused the variance. Variances can be caused by the patient, individual clinical or health care professionals, or because of a fault in the system. When variances to the clinical pathway occur, documentation shows that the variance occurred and what was done to correct the variance at the time. If variances are a result of complex causes, an interdisciplinary case consultation can be convened to discuss the events. The meeting should focus on determining whether the pathway is realistic for the individual patient, as well as whether the variance can be resolved.

Many times, issues arise that were not known when the pathway was implemented, or the patient's condition may have changed since the pathway was started. A patient who is on a fractured hip pathway may develop variances when a comorbid condition, such as hypertension, complicates the treatment. In this case, the treatment would focus on treating the hypertension, since uncontrolled hypertension is life-threatening. The pathway for the treatment of the hip would need to be suspended until the hypertension is controlled, and a hypertension clinical pathway may be implemented. Once this is accomplished, the patient's care can return to the hip pathway. Often, care for both conditions, or any others, can proceed simultaneously.

Decision Trees

Decision trees are used to select the best course of action in situations where there are no clear decisions. Many businesses use decision trees to help them estimate how to determine inventories. An example is a manufacturing company that must decide how much inventory to build before knowing precisely what the demand will be. In the legal industry, an example is a person who must choose between accepting an out-of-court settlement or risk the outcome of a trial. In health care, professionals must also make decisions without complete information. Decision-tree programs allow for the available information to be inputted into a program that systematically factors all variables so that a decision can be made. Many IT systems feature decision trees as part of standard software.

Standards of Care

Standards of care help to operationalize patient care processes by providing a baseline for quality of care delivered to the patient. An example would be a standard that was universally accepted regarding the care of a patient with chest pain. This standard would allow professionals across the country to have an accepted way to systematically treat those patients who suffer from chest pain.

Frequently, standards of care focus on a particular discipline. This gives the professional involved in the treatment a standard by which to practice. The *Standards for Practice for Case Management*, published by CMSA, is an example of professional standards. These standards set forth professional opinions regarding excellence in the field of case management. The standards serve to articulate the role and function of case managers to the public. The public also benefits from establishing standards, as they act to assure quality in practice, perspective, creditability, and legitimacy to the practice of case management. Different disciplines have their own standards to serve as guided, appropriate interactions within their respective practices. The ANA cites standards for nursing care and practice; the AARC cites standards for respiratory care management; the NASW cites standards for social work case management, and so on.

Screening Tools

The general concept of managed care is to educate individuals about how to improve their health status, and to prevent or manage chronic illness, to improve quality of life, and to better control health care costs. To do this, health care professionals must understand how individuals view their own health status, comply with prescribed regimens, perform activities of daily living, and understand individuals' perceptions about quality of life. As a result, health plans and providers must seek valid methods of assessing health status of specific populations and respond to the need to identify at-risk members, to require clinical outcomes accountability, and to focus on population health management.

Health assessment screening tools can be useful in gathering this information. Health assessment screening tools allow providers to proactively evaluate a patient's perception of his/her health status, and whether the patient understands the information given to him/her about a disease or injury, and the ongoing prognosis. After information has been given to a patient regarding a particular treatment or condition, a health assessment screening tool enables the practitioner to evaluate whether the patient understands, and can apply, the information to maximize patient compliance. If the screening tool shows that the patient did not understand the information well enough to self-manage and achieve optimal results, referral to case management is indicated for reinforcement and monitoring the patient's compliance and outcomes over time.

Health assessment screening tools are an effective means to evaluate risk and outcomes. They cannot be used to evaluate process of practice. The methods by which health assessment screening tools are implemented and used should be understood by the case manager, as well as by any member of the health care team using a health assessment screening tool.

Screening tools can be descriptive, predictive, or evaluative.[12] A descriptive assessment tool collects data about the characteristics of a population, to identify and implement health prevention in areas of greatest need. HCFA's *Health of Seniors Measurement* is an example of a descriptive assessment tool used to address risk areas for the frail elderly.[13]

Predictive tools are used to infer what may happen in a particular population, in particular disease conditions, or because of certain lifestyle behaviors. A predictive screening tool may be used to demonstrate factors among smokers. Results would show that smokers tend to develop more respiratory infections and chronic bronchitis than nonsmokers, and recover more slowly from surgery.

Evaluative tools are survey tools that measure and weigh the effectiveness of a particular medical intervention or process. An example would be a screening tool to measure outcomes of diabetic teaching to a population identified by a managed care organization, using a disease management model.[14]

When developing screening tools, an interdisciplinary team that includes physicians is needed. The focus is on establishing and maintaining a streamlined process to make periodic health assessments a routine part of the care process, in both the inpatient and ambulatory settings. The most common screening tool used by providers and managed care organizations is the SF-36. This tool was developed by the Medical Outcomes Trust to survey health status, and which can be used in clinical practice, research, health policy evaluations, and general population surveys. The SF-36 measures eight key points:

- Physical functioning;
- Social functioning;
- Role limitations due to physical problems;
- Role limitations due to emotional problems;
- Mental health;
- Energy/vitality;
- Pain;
- General health.[15]

Examples of other health assessment screening tools that focus on disease- specific care are:

For angina:
1. ROSE questionnaire;
2. Seattle Angina Questionnaire.

For arthritis:
1. Arthritis Impact Measurement Scale (AIMS).

For cancer:
1. Functional Living Index of Cancer.

For mental status:
1. Basis-32;
2. Hopkins Symptom Checklist;
3. Mini-Mental State Examination.

For pain:
1. McGill Pain Questionnaire;
2. MOS Pain Measures.[16]

The impact of health assessment is known only when standard screening tools are adopted industry-wide. Until this occurs, interpretation of health data will remain unclear and incomparable resulting in incomplete benchmarking.

REFERENCES

1. Lovern, E. IOM strikes again. *Modern Healthcare*. 2001:1,4:4–6.
2. Shaw, G. Avoiding a costly learning curve. *Managed Care News*. 2001: 234:236.
3. Cassidy, B. HIPPA: understanding the requirements. *The Remington Report*. 2001: 22, 1:24–26.
4. Simpson, R. Automated outcomes management. In Cohen E, ed. *The Outcomes Mandate: Case Management in Health Care Today*. St. Louis,MO. Mosby; 1999: 226–234.
5. Martin, T, Fuller, S. Components of the CPR: an overview. *Journal of American Health Information Management Association*. 1998: 23:10–20.
6. Frahm, L, Hertz, L. Computer across the continuum. In Cohen, E. ed. *The Outcomes Mandate: Case Management in Health Care Today*. St. Louis, Mo. Mosby;1999; 244–255.
7. Case Management Society of America. A guide to benchmarking and best practice terminology. *Best Practice Conference Proceeding Manual*. Little Rock AR. CMSA; 1999; 1–2.
8. MacRae, S. Patient–centered care: an interview with Susan MacRae. Available at: http://ww1.best4health.org
9. Llewellyn, A, Moreo, K. *Essentials of case management: tools, techniques, principles and practices in case management*. Miramar, FL. Professional Resources In Management Education, Inc.; 1998; 65–66.
10. Pozgar, G. *Legal Aspects of Healthcare Administration*. Gaithersburg. MD. : Aspen Publications; 1993; 516–517.
11. Jackson, R. Guidelines for clinical practice. *British Medical On-line Journal*. Available at: *www.bmj.com*
(12,13,14) Ringel, M. Implementing health status measurement. *Medical Management Network, Strategic Tools for Implementing Evidenced Based Care*. 1998: 6,1:1–16.
15. Ware, J. SF-36 update. *SPINE*. 2000: 25,24:3130–3139.
16. Ross, D. Health status: concepts, measures and applications. *Health Stat*: 1997: 1,2:5.

RESOURCE MANAGEMENT

5

At times, the process of case management is successful, not because of a good data management system, not because a comprehensive rehabilitation plan has been accepted by the payer, and not even because of good clinical practice. Success stems from the case manager's inherent ability to be an excellent resource manager.

Resource management is an integral part of the case management process. A literature search reveals that the term, "resource management" encompasses a wide range of definitions, each germane to a specific environment and process. For example, human resource management pertains to efficient use of manpower in business environments, including safety and human rights of personnel in the workplace, and recruitment and job placement of employees. In the rapidly developing information technology area, resource management refers to efficiency of time, software, and budgets. Natural resource management pertains to appropriate use of our world's natural resources.

Resource management in case management is defined as the process of identifying, confirming, coordinating and negotiating benefits and resources for patients, including health care services, products, and direct care.[1] Resource management involves screening for benefits eligibility, negotiating with payers or providers for out-of-benefit coverage for necessary services and products not covered, and identifying and coordinating care, services, and products that are financially possible for the patient/family when no third-party payer exists. Resource management is a goal-oriented approach.

Resource management requires extensive coordination, well known to case managers, because care coordination is an integral part of each step in the case management process. The ANA recognizes coordination as a core component throughout the entire case management process, not just a specific step.

Coordination of resources is challenging for the case manager. Multiple resources are required by the ill or injured patient/family/caregiver, despite the fact that third-party payment may be limited or not available. Services needed may include transportation, meal preparation, housekeeping, home maintenance, housing, shopping, financial and legal assistance, and regular social interaction, all of which are not covered by most policies because they are considered custodial services. Some payers, such as workers' compensation, cover these services if they are deemed medically necessary.

The process of resource management begins when the case manager completes an assessment of the patient. Collection and recording of comprehensive patient information, is an opportunity to identify specific problems that must be addressed. For example, assessment of the following key areas allows the case manager to identify patient resources:

- Health status
- Functional status
- Psychosocial status
- Cognitive function and mental health
- Medication regimen
- Living conditions and social situation

- Support system
- Compliance or noncompliance with treatment plan(s)

Based on this information, the case manager determines the acuity level of the patient and defines specific goals for the patient. How the goals will be achieved, within appropriate timelines, involves resource management. These areas require the case manager to fully understand the behavioral aspects of the patient/family, requiring social workers to perform resource management for patients in acute care settings. Social workers, as resource managers in inpatient facilities, perform these functions:

- crisis intervention;
- psychological, psychosocial counseling;
- financial assistance assessment; implementation of potential federal/state social service eligibility and application (SSDI, Medicaid, Vocational Rehabilitation, Medicare);
- eligibility determination for support organizations (such as United Way);
- system-wide consultation regarding advance directives, power of attorney, guardianship, placement, etc.

Excellent resource management allows the case manager to be successful in moving the patient toward maximum wellness, and gives the case manager a "feel good" attitude toward his or her role and relationship with the patient. However, resource management can also be time-consuming, frustrating, and limiting in positive outcomes. Lack of community resources, insufficient provider support, and inconsistent family intervention are a few of the common barriers to resource management. For case managers to avoid unnecessary stress and burnout, they must view success as helping patients achieve progress. Therefore, the case manager should balance time spent on resource management with other components of the case management process. The case manager should have a reliable list of current community resources available for continuous reference to reduce stress and maximize efficiency. Networking with other case managers and health care professionals will help the case manager to build resources. Case managers are encouraged to participate in local professional meetings and regional chapter groups of national professional organizations, such as the ANA, SNA, CMSA, or NASW, all of which all have local chapters across the country. A case manager's knowledge base in resource management will continue to grow as he/she matures in the role.

COMMUNITY RESOURCES

Resource management includes many identified goals that will not be covered by the patient's reimbursement system (if any), but can be achieved through use of community resources. The five examples below involve using community resources. The examples purposefully focus on a variety of age groups and challenges to illustrate that community resources can be used for patients of all ages who have disease/injury processes. Each example involves interventions requiring the case manager to obtain prior approval from the patient, and require cooperation from the patient to achieve success. Resource management is part of the overall plan of care developed collaboratively by the case manager, the resource manager (if a distinct role), and the patient/family.

- Goal: Improve nutritional status. The case manager/resource manager may arrange for a nutritional consultation for the patient. He/she may contact the Salvation Army or Goodwill Industries to arrange donation of a microwave oven, and then educate the patient about purchasing easy-to-prepare, nutritionally balanced microwave meals. The case manager/resource manager may arrange for Meals on Wheels or another appropriate social nutritional support service for the patient. Home grocery shopping with a local supermarket may be arranged enabling the patient to phone-in a grocery list and have it delivered weekly.

- Goal: Eliminate threat of patient abuse in home environment. The case manager/resource manager educates the patient regarding an appropriate social service agency in the area to contact, such as Women In Distress, and role-play with the patient to help the patient to understand how to use the agency. The case manager/resource manager may contact the agency to discuss and arrange follow-up intervention strategies by the agency. The case manager/resource manager may identify community outreach centers through a local hospital or high school, where the patient is eligible to participate in classes to develop self-care responsibility. The case manager's responsibility to report abuse will be covered in Chapter ten.
- Goal: Reduce risk of falls in the home. The case manager/resource manager identifies an environmental access specialist in the area who can perform an affordable assessment of the home to eliminate hazardous conditions. Cost-effective solutions include removal of throw rugs or installation of grab bars in the patient's bathroom. The case manager/resource manager also educates the patient and the family/caregiver about medication side effects, such as hypotension as well as polypharmacy risks, and how to prevent side effects, such as rising slowly from a bed or chair. The case manager educates the patient about purchasing an emergency alert system, particularly if the patient has an existing alarm system in the home.
- Goal: Arrange transportation to oncologist's office for chemotherapy. The case manager/resource manager contacts the patient's church or synagogue to request transportation assistance from this community when the patient is too weak to drive himself/herself. The case manager/resource manager contacts the oncologist's office to discuss the patient's fatigue-induced hindrance to driving, and suggests that the physician consider medication or treatment changes to reduce the fatigue. The case manager/resource manager suggests to the patient that he/she schedule oncology visits in the early morning when fatigue is not apparent. The case manager contacts transportation providers in the community who will provide temporary transportation free of charge or on a sliding scale, or explore eligibility to participate in free transportation services provided by the community for disabled individuals. More information on transportation providers is addressed later in this chapter.
- Goal: Improve medication adherence. The case manager/resource manager contacts a reliable family member, friend, or neighbor to set up daily visits or calls to the patient. The case manager/resource manager educates the family member, friend, or neighbor about medication use, how to identify noncompliance, and how to report any problems that arise. The case manager educates the patient about keeping a personal diary to track medication use and various medication treatments. The case manager/resource manager investigates affordable adherence systems, such as a beeping medication reminder system that the patient wears on the wrist, or a more economical oral medication organizer.

The above goal interventions are examples of how the case manager/resource manager can use community resources to aid resource management. In fact, community resources are important components to ensure successful resource management outcomes.

Voluntary Organizations

When community resources are a fundamental component of resource management, volunteer organizations are a fundamental component of community resources. Case managers wishing to ensure successful resource management must have a reliable list of voluntary organizations close to where patients live. Finding volunteer organizations and pertinent contact information is achieved in a variety of ways. National support groups encompass care for major illnesses and injuries, such as the American Heart Association and the National Brain Injury Association. These support groups are accessed on the Internet, via national toll-free numbers, and through local chapters. Major non-profit organizations, such as The Red Cross and The United Way, provide extensive lists of smaller volunteer organizations available in the local area which are usually printed in educational pamphlets intended for consumers. Hospital emergency rooms keep similar lists as resources for patients, and may include support groups germane to the hospital system not otherwise listed in consumer resource pamphlets. Religious organizations are excellent sources of such lists, and include interdenominational organizations that may not be found on other resource lists. The Internet is quickly becoming a resource of choice, although the global nature of Internet resources makes it difficult to identify volunteer organizations focused within one geographic area.

Social Services

Social service agencies are an excellent resource for the case manager, but usually require the patient to meet certain eligibility criteria not required by volunteer organizations. Social service agencies are financed by county, state, and federally matched funds, and therefore not usually as flexible or timely in meeting individual needs as voluntary organizations are. However, social service agencies provide more intense services over a longer period of time. Examples of social service agencies that can assist the case manager to obtain community resources for patients' are: Centers for Independent Living (CIL), area state-run Vocational Rehabilitation offices, and local Area Agency on Aging offices. Case managers should maintain logistical information on area social service agencies, including basic eligibility criteria, office(s) where application for assistance can be made, the qualifying waiting period, if any, and other pertinent information. Some case managers request and keep a supply of eligibility forms for potential patients' use. For example, a case manager covering the obstetrics unit of a hospital will have WIC (Women, Infants & Children) program information on hand to assist a new mother who is financially insecure to obtain free formula for her newborn.

Public Health Services

Public health services are broadly defined as clinical and social services provided by government funding and available to any citizen within the stated geographic area. Examples include public health nurses who visit new mothers to check on the health status of babies and teach new mothers necessary skills, such as safe infant bathing and breast feeding, and outpatient health clinics available in most counties. These clinics have on staff primary care physicians and nurse practitioners, who provide community-sensitive services that are free, or offered on a sliding pay scale, to anyone walking through the door. Primary health care includes medical care, dental care, mental health services, well-child immunizations; adult inoculations to prevent community-acquired diseases, such as influenza and pneumonia; and birth control products/services. Community outreach classes are usually offered on a continuing basis, and provide information about smoking cessation, weight loss, dangers of drug use/abuse, and communicable diseases.

CONSULTATIVE SERVICES

In addition to having a comprehensive list of available community resources, case managers performing resource management consult with other health care professionals to determine available and appropriate services for a patient/family. These professionals may include the attending physician, a home care nurse, therapists, a pharmacist, a social worker, public health nurses, and pastoral care. The case manager performing resource management needs to identify consultative services available in the area.

Consider the 70-year-old male patient admitted to the hospital for a concussion because of an automobile accident. When the case manager is arranging for the patient's discharge to home, he/she learns that the patient's wife is frightened regarding her husband's determination to continue driving. She believes her husband places himself and others at risk because of slowed reflexes and failing eyesight. She states that as his passenger, she has witnessed near-accidents and is fearful of his desire to continue to drive. The case manager speaks to the patient's attending physician, who states that there is no residual neurologic deficit to prevent the patient from driving. The case manager learns that the patient has a valid driver's license that will not expire for another three years.

The case manager speaks to the patient at length about his accident, relays the physician's opinion, and his wife's concerns, and offers information about a voluntary driving evaluation that would ensure his ability to operate a vehicle safely. The patient agrees to the driving evaluation. The case manager then contacts a consultant in the area who is trained to perform driving evaluations for injured/ill individuals. A fee is negotiated that is affordable for the patient, and a driving evaluation is scheduled for two days following hospital discharge.

In many states, patients who sustain head injuries are required to obtain authorization from a neurologist and/or have a driving evaluation before their driver's licenses can be reinstated. In workers' compensation systems, patients involved in different types of injuries undergo driving evaluations as part of their routine treatment plan. Although the case manager in the above example is not in a position to require the patient to receive a driving evaluation, there may be success in convincing the patient to voluntarily seek the evaluation, based upon readily available information about a driving consultant in the area.

Free consultative services are often available through voluntary and social service organizations. Even if a fee is required, these services can be accessed and used to advantage by patients/families. Having information available, when the patient/family needs the consultation, allows the case manager to carry out successful resource management.

VIATICAL SETTLEMENTS

At times, a patient's needs are so expensive that available funds and third-party coverage are not sufficient to pay for services. This financial dilemma created the need for viatical settlements several years ago. Viatical settlements allow companies to purchase life insurance policies from terminally ill individuals with a cash settlement, usually a negotiated portion of the face value of the policy (generally 50–70%). By selling the life insurance policy, the "viator" (the owner of the life insurance policy) is able to obtain a significant portion of the death benefits while still alive, and have available cash to pay for expensive medications, treatments, mortgage/rent, food, or even a dream vacation.

When the viator sells the policy to a viatical settlement company, the company retains ownership of the policy and the beneficiary rights. The company then assumes responsibility to pay the premiums until the person's death, at which time the company collects the full face value of the policy. How much the company will pay the viator at the time of sale of the policy is largely determined by the life expectancy of the viator; a person with six months of life expectancy may be offered 70% or more of the policy's face value, while a person with one year's life expectancy will likely be offered less.

Originally designed for the HIV/AIDS population prior to the advent of HAART (highly active anti-retroviral therapy), when the prognosis of the AIDS patient was much more bleak, viatical settlements as financial resources are now offered to frail, older patients, and to patients with terminal cancer or other terminal illnesses. While viatical settlements offer patients and families a viable means of accessing funds, the decision to accept a viatical settlement may have significant implications. The cash settlement could compromise existing Medicaid or social security benefits[2], or have significant income tax ramifications. The patient/family considering a viatical settlement is making a critical decision at a time that is extraordinarily difficult.

As ethicist Dr. John Banja (1997, 39) notes, "Because viatication frequently occurs in stressful situations during which potential viators may be psychologically vulnerable, providing them with practical and accurate information cannot be overemphasized. "

This information includes offering patients and families alternatives to viatical settlements. One alternative to viatical settlements is an *accelerated death benefit*. An accelerated death benefit allows the life insurance policy owner to surrender the policy by accepting a cash settlement from the company that is less than the face value of the policy at the time of death. Other alternatives include personal loans, cash advances on credit cards, or liquidating assets including real estate or personal property.[3] In addition to offering the patient/family alternative ideas to access funds, the case manager/resource manager should encourage the patient and family to seek financial and/or legal advice, and to receive multiple bids if a viatical settlement is being considered.

Key terms

Viator—terminally ill individual who has an interest in selling his/her life insurance to a third party

Viatical broker—a facilitator who assists the viator in selling the policy

Viatical provider—the funding source who purchases the policy from the terminally ill individual

Viatical settlement—A policy lump-sum settlement available for individuals with an abbreviated life expectancy (often less than 8 years)

Accelerated death benefits (ADB)—benefits available on some life insurance policies and paid to individuals with a life expectancy of approximately 6–12 months. The benefit must be a part of the policy prior to the individual becoming terminally ill.

Viatical online resources

www.viaticaladvocate.com
www.idealsettlements.com
www.viatical-expert.net

SUPPLIES AND EQUIPMENT

Among the ongoing, often expensive resources required by chronically ill/injured patients are the needs for medical equipment and supplies. Medical equipment and supplies, including durable medical equipment (DME), are available from vendors, home medical equipment companies, home health care agencies providing home medical equipment, and retail pharmacies. Other providers include social service and volunteer organizations, hospital therapy and outpatient departments, long-term care and nursing home facilities, and consignment shops specializing in second-hand equipment.

Home medical equipment and supplies can be broadly classified into the following groups of products:

- Ambulation aids, such as walkers, canes, and crutches;
- Bathing and toileting aids, such as shower chairs, tub lifts, hand-held showers, raised toilet seats, and grab bars;
- Respiratory equipment, such as oxygen concentrators, cannulas, masks, nebulizers, peak flow monitors, and pulse oximeters;
- Beds, such as manually adjusted or electric beds, mattresses, and trapeze bars;
- Physical therapy equipment, such as treadmills, stationary bikes, weights, tens units, and CPM (continuous passive motion) machines
- Wound care equipment, such as low air loss mattresses and wound care dressings;
- Enteral products, such as nutrition pumps, tube feeding/oral nutritional supplements, and gastostomy feeding tubes;
- Wheelchairs and accessories, such as manual and power wheelchairs, seat cushions, and storage compartments;
- Personal assistive products, such as reachers, glucose monitoring devices, blood pressure monitors, and portable ramps.

If the needed equipment and supplies require payment from the patient, the amount required is determined by the provider and by the patients' benefits coverage. The case manager engaged in resource management needs to know the best way for the patient to obtain necessary medical equipment and supplies. If health insurance is available, what are the limitations/benefits of coverage for medical equipment and supplies? If the patient has insurance but coverage does not provide for a mattress overlay, can the case manager demonstrate for the insurance company a potential cost savings through prevention of bed sores? If the patient has Medicaid or Medicare coverage, what equipment/supplies are authorized, and who are the authorized area dealers? Is the patient a candidate for a free wheelchair from agencies providing free equipment, such as the Paralyzed Veterans' Association? Is the patient eligible for equipment and supplies through county elder services or public health funding? Is the child a candidate to receive equipment and supplies through Children's Medical Services? If no resources are available, can the patient's physician recommend a less-expensive or alternative type of equipment or supplies?

When deciding who will provide medical equipment and supplies, case managers who are paid by a third party, contact three providers to complete a bid process. All providers must receive the same information, which allows bids to be uniform, and enables the case manager to make an educated decision. All bids should be completed in writing; a verbal quote can be given initially, but should be followed up in writing to assure accuracy.

The case manager includes the following information when requesting a bid. These guidelines should be used even when the case manager is seeking resources from a charitable or reduced-pay resource.

- Specific item or service requested
- Date service or equipment is needed
- Duration of services or equipment needed
- Date and time bid needs to be delivered.

All providers of medical equipment and supplies should be judged on the same criteria that include but are not limited to:

- able to deliver and service equipment and/or supplies;
- have a follow-up plan regarding equipment or service problems;
- describe the type of supervision to be provided;
- instruct about, and support, equipment once ordered;
- have a reputation for dependability and quality of service.

The case manager requests additional contract features that will be in the best interest of the patient, regarding the amount of time the patient is expected to need the equipment/supplies, and whether changes in the patient's physical needs are expected. For example, the pediatric case manager explores options for trade-ins on equipment when the patient grows and needs a larger wheelchair or bed; or a rent/purchase option can be negotiated for the pediatric asthma patient whose long-term use of a nebulizer is uncertain at the time the nebulizer is rented. The case manager should also ask the provider to include the company's return policy on the contract bid. If the pediatric case manager's patient is a wheelchair-bound 14 year old who is likely to begin driving lessons at the age of 16, the case manager will want to explore contract options for future add-on equipment, such as a wheelchair lift. Another contract add-on that should be explored is a service contract, especially if the equipment will be used or is expected to have useful life beyond the manufacturer's warranty period.

Sometimes case managers enter into a case that has been ongoing for some time. Because large expenditures are occurring, the payer or the provider of service identifies the need for case management at a later time in a patient's disease process. The case manager's goal is to reduce costs and maximize available resources, while ensuring the delivery of appropriate, quality care. The pediatric case manager knows that chronically ill/injured children will likely need services over a lifetime. If the case manager enters into an ongoing case, it is important to assess all types of DME equipment currently being used by the patient, and how the equipment is being provided. In one pediatric case, an oxygen concentrator and suctioning equipment had been rented for more than a year. Unaware that they had expended more in monthly rental fees than the cost of purchasing this equipment outright, the insurance company continued to pay fees to a DME provider on a monthly basis. The case manager was able to negotiate a significantly reduced purchase price from the provider, saving benefit dollars for the patient that could be used elsewhere.

Once all contract information is gathered from providers, the case manager determines who will bid on the service or equipment. If all things are equal (quality, service, delivery), the order will likely go to the lowest bidder. If not, the case manager should determine who will be best able to provide the service or equipment, taking into account any financial hardship that may be placed on the patient/family. This decision is summarized with the rationale documented. The case manager may disclose the results of the bidding information to the providers after the contract is awarded, but this is at his/her manager's discretion.

When ordering medical equipment/supplies for a patient, the case manager should follow up to ensure that the equipment is delivered in good working order, and the patient and family/caregiver is comfortable operating the equipment or using the supplies. Additional teaching/training may be required to ensure the patient's safety/health and to prevent an unnecessary hospital re-admission.

The patient and family/caregiver should have information about the equipment agreement that accompanies each piece of equipment. This information includes how the equipment is to be maintained, and the responsibility of the user to maintain the equipment. The patient and family/caregiver are provided with contact information from the equipment manufacturer, and from the agency or company providing the equipment, in case of equipment failure or maintenance is required.

Oxygen

A resource often required by is portable oxygen in the home. Supplemental oxygen is used to maintain adequate tissue oxygenation, using minimal energy by the heart and lungs. The objective is to prevent or correct an abnormal condition in which oxygen available to the body's cells is inadequate to meet the body's needs. Oxygen is considered a drug. As such, the minimal amount of dose required to obtain the appropriate oxygenated response should be prescribed by the physician. An appropriate dose of oxygen will:

- decrease the work of breathing;
- prevent abnormal deficiency of oxygen in the blood;
- decrease excessive work by the heart;
- decrease high pressure in the pulmonary artery.[4]

The case manager needs to understand, and to explain to the patient/family, the minimal dosage required to obtain the appropriate oxygenated response. A problem that can occur if the COPD patient or the acute asthma patient "turns up" the home oxygen supply to feel better, but receives excessive oxygen as a result. Case managers must ensure that patients understand that too much oxygen distorts the respiratory response. Since the body requires a certain amount of carbon dioxide to stimulate breathing, too much oxygen can distort this delicate balance and cause the patient to have respiratory arrest.

Home oxygen is variable in its packaging and portability. Oxygen concentrators are electrically powered and are the most widely used oxygen supplier in the home. Oxygen concentrators are the most cost-efficient means of supplying oxygen to individuals who require continuous home oxygen at low liter flows. Another method of delivery is portable oxygen cylinders, which can be conveniently used with rolling pull-carts for temporary use. They come in various sizes to meet the portable needs of the patient. Liquid oxygen systems provide large quantities of oxygen at low pressures. Portables can be filled from reservoirs for up to an eight-hour supply, at two liters per minute. This makes it valuable for rehabilitation, travel, transport, work, and social outings.

Case managers coordinating oxygen therapy in the home must realize the critical importance of specific patient/family/caregiver education as part of resource management. Oxygen use in the home can be hazardous. Although oxygen is nonflammable, it greatly accelerates the rate of combustion. Oxygen is a colorless, odorless, transparent, and tasteless gas that occurs in nature. Safe use of oxygen demands that all flammable materials and potential ignition sources be removed from the area where oxygen is used or stored.

The case manager will ensure that a knowledgeable clinician provides education and training to the patient/family/caregiver receiving oxygen in the home for the first time. Often, this is a respiratory therapist who may make an initial visit to the home to set up the equipment and ensure its appropriate therapeutic delivery, or who may be authorized for regularly scheduled respiratory therapy visits for the patient. The therapist can also be a trained delivery technician who initially sets up the oxygen equipment/supplies and instructs the patient and family or caregiver to use the equipment and supplies. The person may also be the case manager performing resource management, or the case manager in the payer setting. What is important is that education and training occur with the patient, the family residing in the home, and the caregiver(s) who will be assisting with the oxygen therapy. Education must also be ongoing; any barriers to education must be documented and resolved; and the person(s) delivering the education must have the training and education necessary to instruct the patient/family/caregiver. Education includes teaching the family/caregiver to clean filters to ensure the machine's efficiency, and on how to minimize asthmatic triggers in the home of a child with asthma, such as keeping windows closed or using allergy-free bedding. Key safety features to discuss with the patient/family/caregiver regarding oxygen therapy include:

1. Post no-smoking signs on the front door of the home so that everyone who enters knows oxygen is used. Signs should also be posted in the room in which the oxygen is used or stored.
2. Relocate or remove flammable materials from the area where oxygen will be used, including cotton, wool, polyester fabric, bed clothing, paper materials, plastics, and certain lotions or salves, such as petroleum jelly.
3. Learn and teach others in the home that the most common potential ignition sources are smoking materials, sparks from electrical equipment, or static electrical discharge.
4. Inspect the home or area for these safety tips before placing oxygen in the area.[5]

Disposables

Another product category in resource management are disposables. Disposables include a wide array of products for perineal care and skin care, such as ostomy supplies, wound care, syringes for diabetes, and protective wear for incontinence. Because the use of these products can be life-long, the case manager will carefully compare prices of disposables, and use negotiation skills to create the best agreement that delivers quality, on-time, appropriate products for the patient, while being cost-effective and fiscally manageable.

Many factors must be considered when choosing incontinence products, or when beginning, altering, or changing a bowel and bladder program. Decisions about how to care for the incontinent person are based on many factors, such as:

- The comfort of the incontinent person in using certain products or applying a certain bowel/bladder routine;
- Ease of use by the caregiver;
- Availability of products;
- Affordability of products;
- Durability of products (to minimize accidents);
- Odor control.[6]

Moisture-barrier skin protectors come in a variety of styles and packaging, but are usually available in creams or ointments. Most are long acting and effective in preventing skin breakdown. Cleansers for the perineal skin area are usually available in foam and spray forms and include pH-balanced ingredients for added skin protection. Nonalcohol-based liquid copolymer films are best for individuals who have ongoing incontinence with skin breakdown. Applied to the skin every 12 to 24 hours, they act as a barrier to external moisture and skin irritants, while allowing air to reach the skin to enhance proper skin care. Skin barrier powders are used in conjunction with moisture-barrier ointments for the person who has a stoma. When the powder is applied around the stoma, it dries the skin and allows for an effective "stick" of the moisture-barrier ointment. Underpads are designed to provide maximum absorption away from the skin. Underpads come in different styles and can be worn comfortably with adhesive strips for undergarments, with elastic straps, and with Velcro fasteners.

PHARMACEUTICALS

A changing paradigm in resource management is the use of pharmaceuticals to provide direct-to-consumer education regarding medication compliance and adherence. Only in recent years have pharmaceutical companies engaged in teaching the general public consumer awareness of drug choice. Television ads, print advertising, billboards, and radio announcements are some of the media used by pharmaceuticals to deliver their messages to the public. Sophisticated educational websites specifically geared to the consumer are offered by most pharmaceuticals. This "education campaign" is part of a drug-state-management initiative undertaken by pharmaceutical companies who believe that educated consumers will advocate for, and demand, certain drugs from their primary care and specialist physicians.

Case managers performing resource management can take advantage of pharmaceutical consumer education materials that are a valuable free resource for patients, families, and caregivers, and are a cost-effective, efficient means of providing ongoing medication compliance/adherence education to the patient and family/caregiver. Pharmaceuticals are known to spend thousands of dollars developing educational support documents geared to the individual consumer, free to the consumer and to health care professionals. Available support tools include patient diaries in which the patient is encouraged to write questions to ask the physician at the next visit; care pathways in which the patient is given specific instructions on important nutritional, exercise, functional and psychosocial interventions for a healthy lifestyle; and a myriad of other educationally-based support tools available in user-friendly videos, pamphlets, audiotapes, checklists, books, magazines, and index cards.

Case managers can access a wealth of resource management educational tools by logging onto pharmaceutical companies' websites, and clicking onto the consumer site, or the health care professional site. Several pharmaceutical companies exhibit at national and regional case management conferences, where they display their health care and consumer educational tools. Pharmaceuticals also provide consumer service telephone numbers and health care professional support lines, through which case managers can inquire about available educational materials and access a wide range of resources. These resources serve as professional development tools by allowing the case manager to stay current with available drug therapies, potential comorbid conditions, drug side effects, and symptom management.

The challenge for case managers is to remain objective when accessing this type of provider information. They should also caution the patient to objectively view media advertising and educational pieces regarding prescription and over-the-counter medications. Not every drug is right for every patient. Case managers can encourage the patient to speak directly with his/her physician regarding available drugs and optional treatments.

Some pharmaceuticals also provide patient assistance for those patients who cannot afford the prescribed drug therapy. This includes patients responsible for purchasing their own drugs due to lack of insurance coverage or limited coverage, and those responsible for payment of a portion of their drugs through a co-pay arrangement, and who will require financial assistance in order to receive the prescribed drug therapy. Established criteria to meet eligibility requirements is pre-determined by the pharmaceutical. A sliding-scale payment system is provided by some drug companies, utilizing pre-established criteria to determine the economic needs of patients as well as availability of other assistance.

TRANSPORTATION

A continuing challenge to resource managers is coordinating transportation for patients. Few payer systems finance transportation for the ill or injured individual. Workers' compensation and vocational rehabilitation are two payer systems that have benefit coverage for transportation needs. Some social service systems available for children and the elderly provide transportation and will be discussed in this chapter. Case managers frequently must search for ways to transport a patient who cannot drive himself/herself.

Inability of a patient to drive himself/herself may stem from the patient's illness or injury. This deficit may be a temporary inconvenience for the patient and family, or an adjustment to a debilitating illness or injury that will prevent the individual from driving for a lifetime. The case manager evaluates individual needs of patients. For example, if a patient's physician has prescribed pain medication, and the prescription drug insert information states, *Do not operate heavy machinery while taking this medication*, the patient should not be driving a car while taking the medication. The patient with a fractured right foot should not be driving with the left foot. The oncology patient receiving regular chemotherapy may be too fatigued to drive to the physician's office, missing necessary treatments. Patients may not have had reliable transportation before the illness or injury, and the problem becomes magnified when visits to therapy or to the doctor's office are required.

There may also be times when the case manager will need to assess potential safety hazards for a patient suffering a recent deficit, such as a head injury or stroke patient. As stated earlier in this chapter, the case manager may then need to consider recommending a driving evaluation for the patient by a qualified driving evaluator. In this case, temporary transportation will need to be arranged for the patient, which may result in the need for permanent transportation assistance.

Therefore, there will be many times and many reasons why transportation must be arranged for patients as part of the resource management process. Transportation is available in a variety of systems in most areas of the country, and can be for-hire, not-for-hire, ambulatory or nonambulatory, and private, public, or brokered.

For-hire transportation means that the transporter is able to accept payment directly from the individual. A common example of for-hire transportation is a taxi company. Taxi companies are generally convenient, available, and able to be accessed with little or no pre-planning. However, case managers should be aware that taxi companies dispatch vehicles on an occurrence basis, meaning that the patient can be at the mercy of the dispatch system. Taxi cabs can show up late, early, or not at all. The flexibility of the patient and the flexibility of the appointment should be considered in addition to the cost before accessing a taxi service.

Not-for-hire transportation means that the transporter is not able to accept payment directly from the individual. Rather, payment is made by a third party and is prearranged. Insurance companies commonly use not-for-hire transportation services because it allows the payer to be in direct control of the services the patient is receiving, the charges for the patient's transportation, and the receipt of direct billing. Not-for-hire transportation companies are usually private companies which pre-schedule transportation. These companies usually provide their own contracted drivers.

Some not-for-hire transportation companies are brokered, meaning that they provide administrative coordination for a regional, state or national network of taxi services provided by others. Case managers should exercise caution when using brokered services, as drivers are not directly contracted through the private company, quality cannot be assured, and prices may be higher due to an added layer of brokerage.[7] If a company is advertising nationwide or as extended service, the case manager should inquire regarding the type of direct or indirect services provided by the company.

Case managers are encouraged to call private transportation companies at least 24 hours in advance of services needed for a patient. Generally, the transportation company will require the following information:

- Client's name, address, and phone number (very important)
- Destination site name and address
- Logistical information on who receives the bill
- Information regarding length of time the service is authorized
- Date of injury, claim number and social security number, if the patient is covered under workers' compensation or disability insurance, or;
- Insurance policy number and social security number, if the patient is covered under managed care insurance, or;
- Medicaid or vocational rehabilitation identification number, if any
- Special instructions, such as whether the client uses crutches, a wheelchair or requires other special assistance

Transportation is also classified as ambulatory or nonambulatory. Ambulatory means that the patient can enter and exit a vehicle without assistance. If a company provides ambulatory services, it will be unable to provide special assistance. Many private transportation companies do not provide special assistance because of liability issues. Therefore, if a patient uses a wheelchair, the case manager will need to identify a non-ambulatory company. These are usually listed as wheelchair and stretcher services, and can be either private or public services.

In addition to the private companies, case managers can use public organizations providing special transportation services (STS). These are funded through federal, state, or county funds, or a combination of public funding and private organizational funds. Many STS services require specific patient eligibility. Since preauthorization is required, the case manager will want to encourage and assist the patient in applying as early as possible for services. STS services are usually multi-pickup van services, so the patient will need to allow additional time for transportation to and from the destination. Further, because of the multi-pickup route, there may be a waiting list for services, or inability to provide services to special destinations outside the STS normal route. STS routes often include hospitals, adult day care centers, and other group health settings. Private transportation companies are sometimes contracted for STS services directly through hospital systems.

Sometimes the STS system is the only service available to the patient. The patient should be encouraged to use the system to become familiar with the routes and availability, even if the services may be needed only on an occasional or backup basis. The patient should also be encouraged and assisted to obtain city and county bus schedules and pick-up locations, as well as other public transportation devices, such as trams, rails, trains, and subways. Public transportation is equipped to accommodate wheelchairs and assistive devices; however, the patient must be self-sufficient in order to access public transportation. All public transportation systems have information available on special needs transportation, in accordance with the federal ADA legislation (see Chapter eight), but the consumer may need to request this information. Patients should be educated about the fact that all public transportation systems across the country are required to provide special assistance for the disabled, and to have transportation information readily available in standard print, Braille, and through TDD enhanced hearing services upon request.

Many times, no funding is available to pay for transportation services, and the patient does not qualify for public services. In these instances, resource management can be most challenging. The case manager will need to explore whether there are family members, neighbors, friends, or religious congregation members available to provide volunteer transportation for an ill or injured patient. Unfortunately, organized group volunteer services and even individual assistance are dwindling because of greater awareness of liability and increased litigation. Whenever possible, support transportation should be identified and arranged prior to the time the individual will require assistance.

When a patient's illness or injury causes a permanent deficit that impairs ability to drive, the case manager should explore whether the individual is a candidate to drive with a modified vehicle. Even if the patient is too young to drive, consideration should be given to whether the patient will become a potential driving candidate in the future, and documentation should be provided regarding long-term goals to obtain a modified vehicle for the patient. The case manager strives to achieve the greatest degree of self-sufficiency and independence for a patient. A patient who does not depend upon third-party transportation is achieving a far greater quality of life than one who is dependent upon this system.

An example of a modified vehicle is a van designed to accommodate both a paraplegic driver and the driver's wheelchair. The van's gas pedal, brake, etc., are modified to be operated with hand controls. The side doors are power-operated with a remote, revealing a hydraulic lift for the wheelchair. Additional remote switches activate the lift system and allow the driver to lock his/her wheelchair into the driver's seat position.

While vehicle modifications are expensive initially, they may be far more economical than purchasing transportation services for the remainder of a catastrophically injured person's lifetime. Available funding sources should be considered, including whether the patient has personal access to funding. Some payer systems fund vehicle modification for qualified individuals. These include, but are not limited to, workers' compensation, some group health indemnity plans, and vocational rehabilitation. Companies in the private sector complete vehicle modifications and maintenance/repairs. Most of the major car companies now have programs in place for qualified disabled individuals, whereby vehicle modifications are completed at cost, or free, at the time a new vehicle is purchased.

ASSISTIVE TECHNOLOGY

Assistive technology (AT) is rapidly increasing in availability to assist patients with their activities of daily living. AT are the tools that individuals with disabilities (including the normal aging process) use for living, learning, working and playing.[8] Assistive technology includes any equipment or device that increases the independence of a person with a disability. Wheelchairs, prostheses, visual aids, computers, adapted sports equipment, and augmentative communication devices are all included under the term AT.[9] Without personal assistance devices, many people with physical disabilities would be leading isolated and dependent lives.[10] Therefore, AT is a common classification of products required by ill or injured individuals, and by children and adults with congenital birth defects.

AT can be considered "high tech" or "low tech". Computers are an example of a high technology assistive device, performing a myriad of tasks. Computers can provide communication systems for people with speech disabilities. They can also be used to create a "smart house". Smart house AT systems perform many functions through the individual control of a keypad, including opening/closing doors and windows, adjusting the thermostat, and turning on/off lights. Computers can also be used to play cards, access the Internet, balance a checkbook, plan a menu, or even shop. Computers can be adapted so that they are activated with one large switch, with a mouthstick (blowing into a straw), or with a touch pad to be used by the knee, foot, or elbow.

Other forms of high tech AT include battery operated devices you wear on a wristband. Examples are beeping medication reminder systems, and safety transmitting devices with a panic button to advise others of an emergency situation. High tech AT products also assist disabled individuals in social activities. Examples include special ergonomic tools for gardening, a modified single/double ski for an amputee snow skier, and computerized fishing rods and gun holders.

There are many forms of "low technology" assistive devices. Examples include:

- zipper pulls and Velcro closures on shirts and pants;
- special feeding utensils, such as large-handled utensils for easier grasping, or with weights to decrease hand tremors;

- reachers, which are pick-up tools to reach low and high areas without bending, stooping, or stretching, or that would otherwise be unreachable;
- book holders to assist in holding a book, turning pages, or enlarging letters;
- offset door hinges to make existing doorways wider for a walker or wheelchair;
- grab bars and safety rails, which can be purchased in various lengths and installed near toilets and tubs to assist an individual while toileting or bathing;
- portable ramps to assist an individual or the caregiver in accessing raised areas, such as the front door.

Assistive technology items can be purchased from medication vendors, large retail drug stores, therapy clinics, specialized stores or catalogs, environmental access specialists, assistive technology providers and service specialists, and durable medical equipment companies. Some equipment vendors loan equipment for a certain period of time before requiring a purchase. It is important to work with vendors who are knowledgeable regarding AT products. Appropriate AT products can be adapted to a person's functional needs and capabilities—they should not require the person to adapt to functions and features specific to the device.[11]

REFERENCES

1. Bower, K, Falk, C. Case management as a response to quality, cost, and access imperatives. In E. Cohen ed. *Nurse case management in the 21st century* St. Louis, MO. Mosby; 1996; 161–167.
2, 3. Banja, J. Are viatical settlements ethical? *Journal of Care Management.* 1997: 3,3:33–40.
4, 5. Casteel, B. Use of oxygen in the home. Available at: www.cando.com
6. Moreo, K. The essentials of skin care for incontinence. Available at: www.cando.com
7. Winter, J, Middleman, S. Costly mistakes in transportation: Transporting the injured worker. Liberty Mutual Insurance Company Presentation. Pompano Beach, Fl. 2000.
8, 9. Hobart, K. Assistive technology: What it is and how it can help you. Available at: www.cando.com
10, 11. Scherer, M.J. Assistive technology: A plain english primer. *Case Review.* 1997: 25, 4:79–81.

UTILIZATION MANAGEMENT

6

The overuse of health care resources and its impact on cost first gained the full attention of the health care industry in 1975, when an amendment to the Social Security Act created the Professional Standards Review Organization (PSRO). The purpose of the PSRO committee, as briefly explained in Chapter four, was to involve local practicing physicians in ongoing professional peer review and evaluation of health care services delivered under Medicare. To avoid sanctions by Medicare, hospitals supported PSRO committees as a means to address the appropriateness of services delivered and whether acute care days were justified. Nurses were put into positions to review the same information that the PSRO committee would review if a site inspection were to occur. The goal was to anticipate cases that might be denied or investigated, and work with the doctor to provide necessary documentation to justify services.[1]

The nurses performing the PSRO functions, and the departments created to oversee this process in each hospital, became known as the utilization review (UR) department. Ironically, despite the fact that UR became an active department throughout hospital systems, Congress was dissatisfied with the results. The PSRO was later replaced by PRO. Then, in an attempt to further decrease Medicare costs, Congress enacted the Prospective Pay System in 1983. This measure significantly changed Medicare reimbursement from a fee-for-service system to services reimbursed on a pre-determined fixed price formulated through diagnostic related groups (DRGs). A Medicare pricing formula was established for 492 specific diagnostic categories.

DRGs became a source of huge discussions in UR departments, as well as in the offices of chief financial officers. The financial implications of the DRG payment system caused hospitals to critically look at how care was provided to address long-term financial viability.[2] For the first time, hospitals became accountable to treat patients who fell into a given DRG at a pre-determined cost, despite the length of time the patient remained in the hospital. Hospitals soon identified four primary ways in which costs of a DRG could be reduced:

- Reduce the price paid for resources.
- Reduce the length of stay.
- Reduce the intensity of service provided.
- Improve the efficiency of the service delivered.

Hospital administrators began to analyze how each department was a cost center impacting the total delivery cost of a specific DRG. The UR department played a large role in this determination. UR nurses were pressured to decrease length of stays by taking an active role in the management of resources. They were expected to ensure that any diagnostic test performed on a Medicare patient had a medical reason for being performed. If there was no clear rationale provided in the medical record, the physician who ordered the diagnostic test was questioned regarding its appropriateness. To improve efficiency, if diagnostic tests were not performed in a timely manner, supervisors were held accountable. Further, as soon as diagnostic reports were available in the patients' charts, the UR nurse would call the physician to discuss the results and ask for the next step in the treatment plan.

This change in patient management caused adversarial relationships throughout the entire health-care system, but was justified by administration as a means to remain fiscally viable. Meanwhile, many hospitals took active steps to turn their marketing strategies away from senior citizens in the community and toward the younger insured population. They were headed for a rude awakening.

Commercial insurance carriers were following the direction that Medicare had started, and were beginning to look at the cost of care. Initially, they did this by retrospectively reviewing records, using their own UR nurses to match cost with care. If charges did not match the documentation in the medical record, payment was denied by the payer. In addition to retrospective review, they began sending nurses into hospitals to follow patients while they were hospitalized; or had a payer-based UR nurse call the hospital UR department for an update on the progress/lack of progress the patient was making. If the payer believed that the patient did not meet criteria to remain in the hospital, the physician was pressured to produce documentation to justify the hospital stay. If adequate documentation was not received, payment for a portion of the hospital stay was deducted from the payment. Eventually, this practice also spread to other provider settings, such as home care, skilled care facilities, and post-acute programs.

In time, the industry realized that focusing solely on the cost of care was not the most efficient way to manage resources, and jeopardized quality and continuity of care. Thus, the focus of UR was broadened to focus more attention on utilization management (UM) of resources that would include quality of care and resource allocation in an attempt to improve services, and to reimburse for services.

Today, both payers and providers of health care services have various models, levels, and processes of UM in place to ensure attention is given to resource management, cost effectiveness, and quality. Some blend UM functions into case management; others keep UM and case management as separate and distinct departments. Those professionals who have been involved in the health care industry for some time and witnessed what started as a subtle change, can understand the monumental paradigm shift that has occurred over the years. Those who have recently entered the practice will gain a better understanding as a result of this chapter.

While UM continued to retrospectively address escalating health care costs through the 1980s and early 1990s, the practice of case management was gaining attention as a proactive approach to cost, quality, and access to appropriate services. Many payers were experiencing success when case managers worked with catastrophic patients, and believed that case management could be equally effective for patients with lesser acuity. By assigning patients to case management services early on and addressing their course of care in a proactive fashion, admissions were being avoided, resources were being used less frequently, and patients were reporting greater satisfaction.

Payers and providers alike began to define and redesign a blended model of UM and case management. By integrating principals of UM and case management, providers and payers found that they could independently and collaboratively manage both the benefits and the patients without compromise of one or the other. This occurred using retrospective monitoring of resources used by the majority of plan members through the UM approach, and proactive monitoring of high cost, high acuity plan members through case management.

Further, UM was broadened to include a process still used today—providing a stepping stone into case management. Through the use of ongoing monitoring, patients who have repeat admissions, major setbacks to their care, or social problems that impede adherence or compliance, are triaged by the UM specialist into case management services. The case manager's first role is to develop an individualized care plan that addresses these holistic problems. The ability to do this has evolved further with the sophistication of IT systems that provide risk stratification and patient identification.

As the population ages and scientific advances allow people to live longer, controlling chronic illness and complications inherent to the aging process will become more critical. The emergence of disease management has enabled medical professionals to understand disease processes and to provide specific interventions geared to effectively control disease processes. Blending principles of disease management, utilization management and case management provides payers and providers with a three-pronged approach to patient care management across the continuum of life.[3] The blending of these distinct principles will continue to evolve over time. To keep pace, case managers and other health care professionals are challenged to maintain and enhance clinical competencies. In addition, health care professionals must have a clear understanding of how health care services are reimbursed. The next section will address benefits coverage, while information on disease management will be addressed in Chapter seven.

BENEFITS COVERAGE

As Chapter nine indicates, health care reimbursement systems vary greatly in design and coverage. Utilization managers and case managers must be aware that patients are covered by different variations and types of plans, each with its own rules and limitations. The goal of utilization management is to use the resources covered under an individual benefit plan appropriately, to meet an individual's health care needs.

Assuming that a patient has health insurance, it will be important for the utilization manager and/or case manager to determine the type of plan the patient has, once the plan of care is determined. The type of plan the patient has will determine the scope of services and benefit coverage that will apply. Many times, authorization is needed before services or products can even be ordered. Utilization managers, case mangers, and providers should no longer claim they don't know the rules when it comes to understanding the covered benefits of a specific payer. The payer is obligated to provide information once a request is made, and if this information is not provided in a timely manner, a grievance can be filed. In general, the more "managed" a plan is, the more restrictive the rules to be followed.

The first thing a provider must do when working with a patient from a traditional managed care organization, is to obtain authorization from the primary care physician. This must occur before treatment or services can be provided. Also, it will be important to verify with the payer those providers that are part of the managed care network. Managed care patients must stay within a network of providers to receive care if they want services covered. Utilization managers and case managers should also realize that many patients are unaware of the type of plan or benefits they have, since many times they have not taken the time to read their member handbooks or acquaint themselves with the plan. In addition, due to rising health care premiums, many employers switch plans frequently, so that keeping up with various benefit packages can be a challenge for the average person. Patients may also have a choice to seek services out of the managed care network, but depending upon their plan and the restrictions, products and services may not be covered, or covered only partially; patients will be responsible for the amount not covered.

Consider the repercussions when a physician sends a patient for lab tests to a noncontracted laboratory. Keep in mind that the ideal situation would be for the patient to know which laboratories participate in their insurance plan. Often, the patient is not aware that it is necessary to use a network provider for diagnostic tests. The patient will usually follow the instructions that the doctor or the office staff recommends. Since many doctors participate in various plans and use various diagnostic labs within those networks, referring a patient to the wrong lab can easily occur. It is important for the provider to check, or advise the patient to check with his/her managed care organization or the benefits handbook before seeing a provider, to avoid the following scenario.

The patient goes to a diagnostic lab that is not a part of the patient's insurance network and has the lab work performed. Subsequently, the managed care plan refuses to pay the invoice submitted for lab services performed. Since the lab is not contracted with the managed care plan, the lab seeks payment directly from the patient. Unfortunately, the patient will usually not find out that the lab was not part of the provider network until the bill arrives. The patient calls the laboratory billing department thinking a mistake has occurred. The billing department advises the patient to call the managed care plan to discuss billing questions. The customer service representative at the managed care organization checks the list of network providers and informs the patient that he/she went to the wrong lab. The patient states that the physician's nurse gave him/her the instructions and directions to the lab. The customer service representative at the managed care plan will inform the patient that he/she is ultimately responsible to know what provider to use, not the doctor. This exchange immediately sets up an adversarial situation between the patient, the payer, and the provider. The outcome that will usually occur is that the patient will be responsible for the total bill or a portion of the bill.

This scenario, although frustrating, could be worse if the same patient went to a hospital for surgery, only to find out that the hospital and the surgeon were not in the approved network. A process called pre-certification, which will be discussed later in this chapter, usually avoids this situation before expensive services are rendered.

Utilization managers, case managers, and health care providers have a responsibility to verify benefits for all procedures and services as part of the utilization process. Proactively educating the patient and the family to become familiar with the guidelines of their insurance policy is important, since the patient can be held financially responsible for charges. If the patient does not have the funds to pay the portion for which they are responsible, the provider may go without reimbursement. Many providers and managed care organizations have enhanced UM departments with sophisticated IT systems that enable the precertification process to be more efficient and faster by linking information that allows the UM nurse to process information faster, more consistently and with integration to the medical management process.

An example of this technology is a computer program that has multi-screen applications. These programs create seamless environments so that the utilization manager has the ability to verify enrollment status and benefit coverage for the multitude of members for which he/she is responsible. These systems allow professionals to track medical information, to document medical necessity, review clinical guidelines and pathways, and monitor patients through electronic health records. The systems assist case managers, utilization managers, and providers in ensuring that care is delivered in an organized and timely manner.

DIAGNOSTIC TESTING

Diagnostic testing presents the greatest area where precertification and concurrent review is used. Diagnostic testing procedures are key tools that physicians use to accurately diagnose and screen patients for services. Each physician has his or her own method for determining a working diagnosis for a patient. Essential to making an accurate diagnosis is obtaining a comprehensive history, performing a physical examination, and then deciding which diagnostic procedures need to be used to confirm the preliminary diagnosis. In deciding what tools will be used, physicians choose procedures and tests that have proven validity, are reliable, safe and, when possible, cost-effective.

As this chapter and this book have demonstrated, managed care caused a shift of risk from the payer to the provider. Because of this shift of risk, the potential exists to over- or underutilize diagnostic tests and procedures. To avoid this and ensure that specific diagnostic tests are medically necessary, managed care- based UM specialists require information from the provider to support medical necessity for the procedure.

An example to demonstrate this concept is the case of an orthopedic physician who sees a patient with a back injury. The physician speaks to the patient to determine the cause of the injury, obtains a history, examines the patient, and develops an initial plan of care. The physician may follow a treatment guideline specific to back pain that outlines the course of care. This care may include physical therapy three times a week for four weeks to decrease spasms, and a mild analgesic and an anti-inflammatory medication. On the other hand, if the patient is having periods of incontinence accompanying the pain, the physician will likely order an MRI to rule out cauda equina syndrome, an emergency neurological condition caused by compression of the vertebrae on spinal nerves. The physician will document the complaint of incontinence when he orders the test, to provide the medical necessity for why he went outside the traditional guideline for back pain. On the other hand, if the doctor orders an MRI and has no clear documentation to support the request, the pre-certification utilization specialist is likely to deny the test, since there is no supporting evidence to certify that the test is to be done outside the guideline.

Diagnostic testing can also be used to support medical necessity when procedures and treatments are requested. Diagnostic testing provides evidence that allows the physician to build a case that supports his/her diagnostic impressions. Clear documentation should accompany all requests for service. By providing this documentation in advance, time delays can be avoided and care delivery can be enhanced.

CONTRACT PROVISIONS

For managed care providers to effectively manage risk within a managed care network, providers are selected who can adequately provide services to meet the health care needs of the members. Several factors are taken into consideration when a network considers its list of providers. Providers seeking to join a managed care organization's network must meet certain criteria and standards. Standards may be set by the managed care network, by a state legislative agency if the state mandates that managed care networks exist, or by an accreditation organization. An example of when a state mandates provisions of a managed care network occurs if a state's legislature requires the state workers' compensation division to operate under a managed care system. This is required in many states to control costs. In this scenario, managed care networks are set up to include providers who agree to follow specific mandates set by the state, such as special certification or special training in managed care principles. In addition to following these requirements, the providers may also be required to follow the individual managed care organization's standards. Also required, as part of the contract requirements may be that providers possess certain credentials.

For example, acute care hospitals, home care agencies, and DME companies may need to be accredited by the Joint Commission on Accreditation of Healthcare Organizations (JCAHO), to even be considered as a network provider. Further, the provider's staff must be properly professionally credentialed to ensure quality and appropriateness of the staff for the types of services being delivered. A managed care organization will want to ensure that a provider also has adequate liability coverage.

Once all of the requirements are met for application as a network provider, the managed care organization will ensure that the provider can deliver reports and outcomes that will be needed when the managed care organization undergoes its own continuing accreditation process. This information is important, since the managed care organization is responsible for selecting providers who can provide quality care for their members. One way to prove this is with objective outcomes from the provider. Finally, providers who join a managed care network must agree to the reimbursement rate that the managed care organization offers, which is usually on a capitated basis. The provider is paid a fixed fee that cannot be altered despite how often the provider's services are accessed.

These requirements are necessary to ensure that the providers in the network follow the standards set by the managed care organization and by imposed legislation. Policies and procedures are usually reviewed on an annual basis when provider contracts are renewed. Once a contract is signed, the provider can begin to serve members in the managed care organization. Case managers working with and for providers in a network have a responsibility to monitor the care provided. If care is not up to the expectations of the managed care organization, the case manager can file a grievance against the provider through the quality department within the managed care organization. Likewise, patients can also file grievances against network providers. The managed care organization must address all grievances in writing to members within a specific time frame and note what is being done to address the grievance. Grievances will be covered later this in this chapter.

NETWORKS

The development of provider networks is one of the ways that managed care organizations can deliver quality, cost-effective care for the members they cover. As demonstrated in the prior section, networks are made up of contracted providers who agree to provide services for a group of members within a managed care organization for a negotiated or capitated price. Networks are made up of clinicians and ancillary providers who can provide the range of primary and specialty services needed to meet the needs of the managed care organization's members.

The managed care organization determines the extent, type, specialization, and overall number of providers needed within its network. This formula will change as the organization's members move into and out of its various plans. Usually, a network will contain multiple providers of like services, but will limit the number of like providers based upon the demands and needs of the members who will use the network.

For example, a managed care network may include three large home care agencies, with each providing a full range of high-tech and standard home care services. The network will also include two smaller agencies that cannot provide high-tech care, but are important for members of the plan because they are located in rural areas. Other services a network may provide include diagnostic radiology and laboratory services, durable medical equipment, infusion and pharmaceutical services, respiratory therapy services, and physical/occupational therapy services. Depending on the type of managed care plan, members are required to use network providers when they receive care as directed by the primary care physician. Networks strive to include providers who have an excellent community reputation, are geographically diverse, and can administer all access points of patient care. Network providers are held accountable for the care that they provide and are reviewed on an ongoing basis by the quality department within the managed care organization.

Over- and Underutilization

Network providers agree to accept the financial risk for the services they provide, thus transferring risk from the payer to the provider. Providers who accept financial risk must be cautious not to under- or overutilize services. A home care company that assumes risk to provide home care services for members of a large managed care organization receives a fixed fee per member to provide any home care services assigned. If services are used appropriately, the home care company will be able to budget its funds to cover its costs. If the services are overutilized, the home care agency cannot obtain additional funding to cover additional expenditures.

For the home care agency to ensure proper utilization, all patients who require home care services must be properly monitored. This includes proactive management to ensure that patients are being discharged to home at the right time, and can assume responsibility for their care or have family or community support in place, since home care services will be only temporary. The provider will assign his/her own UM specialist or case manager to monitor the care and the costs associated with the care.

It is important that patients and families receiving services from home care agencies are taught how to perform self-care as soon as possible, so that home care can be safely decreased or discharged. Patient diagnoses and overall conditions will determine ongoing home care needs. If a home care agency determines that two visits are appropriate to teach a patient and the caregiver how to perform dressing changes, it will be important for the agency's UM specialist or case manager to follow-up after the teaching has been given to determine whether the patient/caregiver is able to perform the task as taught. If the patient or caregiver is able to demonstrate comfort and skill with the task, one follow-up visit by a home care nurse may be all that is needed to establish a safe discharge and still make a profit. On the other hand, if the patient and caregiver do not appear capable of performing the task, more visits will be necessary, even if the additional visits are costing the agency money. The provider assumed the risk of caring for the patient when he/she accepted the patient.

Overutilization can cost providers great loss. A fine balance is important to ensure proper use of services. Clinical guidelines and pathways are important tools for UM specialists and case mangers to follow to ensure proper use of services. Information regarding clinical guidelines and pathways is presented in Chapter four. Managed care organizations routinely review providers as part of their continuous quality improvement process. In a review, the managed care organization retrospectively looks at the provider's list of cases to evaluate how services were provided. If the managed care organization's quality team sees evidence of under- or overutilization of services, the provider will be given a warning. If the situation is not corrected in a timely manner, the managed care organization can cancel the provider's network contract.

DENIALS AND APPEAL PROCESS

Managed care has been difficult for many providers and consumers to understand and adapt to over the years. This is mainly because many of the rules and regulations implemented by managed care organizations are viewed as roadblocks to prevent access to needed medical care. The essence of the managed care concept is to provide care to members of an organization in a timely manner using providers who appropriately manage access to care while ensuring quality and cost effectiveness. To comply with this philosophy, managed care organizations will deny a treatment or therapy if the medical documentation of the provider does not support the necessary level of care or service requested.

Provider case managers need to be alert to this, and remember that they hold many of the answers to questions that the managed care organization requires. If the UM department of a managed care organization denies an admission, a day, a treatment, or a procedure, the provider and the patient have a right to "due process", and can appeal the decision. Many states, as well as the accrediting organizations, require managed care organizations to inform members and providers that they have the right to an appeal, and to provide information regarding the appeal process. When an issue arises that the provider or member does not agree with, an appeal can be made to the managed care organization, asking for reconsideration of the decision.

Managed care organizations, as part of their structure, are required to establish policies and procedures to handle both appeals and grievances. Each managed care organization has a department specified to process appeals and grievances. An appeal is a formal method of lodging a disagreement over a claim payment or benefit denial. Once an appeal is filed, the managed care organization is obligated to answer the appeal within a certain period of time. In the case of precertification denials or appeals, the time period to make a decision is shorter. If a provider feels there is an urgent need for treatment and the request is denied, the provider must notify the payer that an appeal is urgent, so that the process can be expedited.

When appealing a claim, it is important that all benefit information be provided, along with medical documentation and with a cost-benefit analysis supporting the need for the service or procedure. Many times, the provider case manager will be the professional who initially files the appeal. The provider case manager should follow the chain of command within the managed care organization. The provider case manger may consult with the medical director of the provider organization, or with the physician who has requested the services, to strategize how to best present the appeal. Many times, having the provider physician speak directly with the managed care organization's medical director will allow a resolution to be achieved through peer-to-peer interaction. It is important that all efforts, specific timelines, and conversations are documented.

In addition to the appeal process within each managed care organization, most states also require an external review process (ERP) to allow consumers and providers an opportunity to challenge the payer's denial of medical coverage.[4] The external review process provides an opportunity to have a third party, independent of the managed care organization, examine the file of a denied claim to render an opinion.[5] To initiate an independent review claim, the provider or patient must have a written notice from the payer that a claim is denied. The information is then turned over to the state insurance commissioner's office and a medical specialist, certified in the health care field pertinent to the denial, will review the claim. The specialist has the authority to determine whether the medical claim should be covered. If the decision is in favor of the claim, the payer must cover the claim.

In addition to the appeals process, managed care organizations are required to set up a process whereby providers and members are able to voice complaints or grievances. A grievance is a formal method of lodging a complaint with the managed care organization.[6] Of note is that grievances can be filed by the managed care organization against a network provider, or by the network provider against the managed care organization, or by a patient regarding the managed care organization and/or the network provider. Grievances are filed when there is a problem or an issue that causes a delay in care, or other care- related issues that the managed care member or provider may have. Some of the reasons that a grievance may be reported include timeliness of claims handling, an unprofessional experience with a network provider, a problem with a provider's office staff, a delay in treatment or service caused by the managed care organization due to the untimely approval of a service, or a product/service that is medically necessary and is not a covered benefit. Filing a written grievance gives the managed care organization a formal opportunity to address the problem and rectify the situation. If a provider or a member takes the time to file a grievance, the managed care organization should respond in writing regarding what action was taken to correct the situation.

AUTHORIZATION AND CERTIFICATION

Utilization management is achieved through prospective, concurrent, and retrospective review techniques. The remainder of this chapter will cover the method by which care and services are reviewed in general terms in a managed care environment. Health care professionals should be aware of each individual payer's UM processes, and follow them as outlined by each organization.

Preauthorization Review

Preauthorization or preadmission review is performed before a service or a product is started. Preadmission review is used to determine the actual need for a patient's admission or treatment as outlined by a specific provider. An example that can illustrate this process is the need for a hip replacement on a 55-year-old female patient with a history of osteoarthritis. The managed care organization's guidelines state that a second opinion for all patients under the age of 65 receiving a hip replacement is required. The rationale for this is that due to the cost of hip replacements, the managed care organization wants to ensure that all conservative measures have been exhausted prior to authorizing a hip replacement. Younger patients traditionally have more options available to them to avoid surgery.

The member is notified of a denial by the UM department's pre-admission nurse, and is given the choice of either seeking a second opinion by an orthopedic surgeon elsewhere in the network, or consulting with his/her physician for alternative treatment. The plan member decides to get a second opinion. If a case manager were involved, he/she would ensure that a written report from the original orthopedic surgeon is available for the second physician at the time of the appointment, along with any x-rays and diagnostic tests that the patient may have had. The case manager ensures that a written report from the physician rendering the second opinion is sent in a timely manner to the original orthopedic surgeon, who then discusses with the patient an appropriate course of action.

UM specialists use various methods to precertify a procedure or product to ensure that it meets criteria. The UM specialist reviews the information submitted, comparing it with the review criteria in his/her precertification computer program. Once this review is done, the specialist renders a determination. If an admission or a procedure is denied, the provider must review the reason for the denial and contact the treating physician or clinician to obtain the necessary documentation that supports the procedure or service. If this is not possible, the provider restructures the plan of care to meet the needs of the patient. If this is not in the best interest of the patient, the provider has the option of an appeal.

Concurrent Review

Concurrent review is a process used to document the continuation of a service that a patient may be receiving, such as a continued hospital stay. It occurs concurrently with the services /products being delivered to ensure that eligibility criteria for the service/product continues to be met. Concurrent review is most common in hospitalizations, care that is provided in a rehabilitation facility, and care delivered by infusion or home care providers.

A managed care organization may require that concurrent review be performed by the provider's UM department on a daily basis, or the managed care organization may complete its own daily or ongoing review of the provider organization. This is often done when criteria for the admission or service are short term, or if care has been continuous for an extended period of time and progress is slow. The provider is challenged to support the level of care that is being requested with adequate documentation. In other cases, where a patient is critically ill and the condition is not expected to change on a day-to-day basis, the review may be performed on a weekly basis.

To develop a professional relationship with the payer UM department, the provider or provider case manager provides reviews that explain the clinical picture in as much detail as possible. It is important to give reports of all diagnostic tests that have been performed and show that they were performed promptly. It is also important to report the response of the patient to any treatments, since this information helps support that the treatment or procedure is helping to meet the outcome of moving the patient toward a lesser level of care.

For example, a patient who is in a rehabilitation facility for therapy related to a head injury may initially be approved for a two-week period. The provider case manger responsible for providing an update to the managed care organization's UM department must show the progress the patient has made, as well as the goals the team feels the patient can achieve with continued effective therapy. Depending on the outcome of the case manager's report, the team will be informed and the plan of care will be continued, or an alternative plan may need to be developed. If the continued stay is denied and the multi-disciplinary team feels strongly that it is in the patient's best interest to remain, objective documentation to support these feelings must be provided. If the request is denied again, an appeal can be made, or the alternative plan can be put into place. Detailed documentation regarding all discussions and documentation should be incorporated into the patient's chart.

Developing a collaborative relationship with the managed care organization's UM specialists is essential so that the provider case manager gains a clear understanding of the criteria the utilization specialist is seeking. Also, by ensuring professional rapport, trust can be established that will aid in better communication and improve the working relationship between the provider and the payer. However, once trust is established, it must be respected. If the provider breaches that trust, working collaboratively on future cases will be very difficult.

Many providers use one set of guidelines, such as Interqual™ for concurrent review, while the managed care organization may use another system, such as Milliman and Robertson. These are just two examples of the many different guidelines used throughout the health care system. Many times, these systems don't "talk" to each other, resulting in conflicting information. Collaboration between the provider and managed care UM specialist becomes paramount to ensure that any miscommunication is resolved prior to a decision being made. Both sides must remember that there is a patient at risk. The provider has the patient in view and must paint an accurate picture to support the treatment. It is also important that the provider is proactive in moving the patient to a lesser level of care as soon as medically stable. Working with the team to move the patient along the continuum is an essential role for the provider case manager. It is critical that the patient and family are kept in the communication loop to update them regarding the plan of care and what is to be expected in the future. Ensuring that the patient and family are part of determining the concurrent plan of care is necessary to achieve success and adherence.

Retrospective Review

A retrospective review is performed after care or service is provided. Retrospective reviews can be viewed as part of the continuous quality improvement process that both the provider and the payer use to improve services. Many managed care organizations have reduced or eliminated the pre-certification process, but are looking retrospectively to see how providers have managed care of members. If a provider is seen as an outlier, which is a provider who either under- or overutilizes services when measured against peers, the managed care organization uses retrospective data to show the provider how he/she compares with other peers having similar patients on a national basis. This process has led to improvement in practice and has also given validation to the use of clinical pathways and patient care guidelines. As discussed in Chapter four, these tools allow providers and payers to have a road map that enables care to be purposeful and timely, and which lowers variance in care. UM specialists and case managers who use these tools as comparison markers in retrospective review must remember that they are meant to be guides, not clinical decision makers. Outlier decisions made by clinicians during a patient's course of care may have valid reasoning based upon a difficult case or unusual circumstances. Retrospective review paints a picture of what occurred, and allows both payers and providers to determine potential changes that can be made to promote continuous quality improvement.

REFERENCES

1. Delong, M. Utilization management: A core course. Available online at: http://cyberchalk.com/nurse/shoppingCart/index_NW.cfm
2. Cleverley, W. *Essentials of healthcare finance*. Gaithersburg, MD. Aspen Publications, Inc.1992; 18–20.
3. Carneal, G. The evolution of utilization management. *Managed Care Interface*. 2000: 24,12: 86–92.
4, 5, 6. AETNA U.S. Healthcare Insurance Healthcare Member Handbook. Hartford, CT. 1999:3–13.

DISEASE MANAGEMENT

7

As demonstrated in the previous chapter, utilization management has caused the health care industry to focus on illness, rather than wellness, for nearly 30 years. Historically, the delivery of health care in the U.S. has focused most of the resources, treatments, and services to address the acute effects of chronic disease. As a result, costs have escalated and outcomes reported have not justified expenditures.

Today, it is known that chronic diseases are major killers and drivers of cost. Chronic diseases are defined as conditions that are prolonged, do not resolve spontaneously, and cannot be cured.[1] Statistics from the Centers for Disease Control and Prevention (CDC) estimate that more than 90 million Americans live with chronic illness, and more than one in five adults are considered disabled from chronic diseases. Further, the direct medical care costs associated with chronic diseases account for more than 60% of the nation's medical care costs.[2] Attempts to control costs are further complicated by the graying of America and numerous scientific advances that have enabled people to survive longer with complex medical conditions.

Employers, payers, and government officials have demanded that the health care industry find a more efficient and effective method to provide health care services. Disease management represents a proactive health care delivery approach that requires day-to-day management of chronic diseases, to minimize or prevent complications or exacerbations that lead to high use of expensive health care services.[3] Disease management allows health care professionals to coordinate care that addresses a specific illness, rather than a particular aspect of treatment, to achieve the best clinical outcomes for an identified patient population in the most cost-effective manner. Case managers, acting as liaison among providers, payers, and patients are integral to a successful disease management program. Case managers promote quality, cost-effective care by implementing the essential functions of case management to identify and address specific health care needs for patients with a particular chronic disease. This chapter will provide insight into various aspects involved in the practice of disease management. Case managers, regardless of setting, can work together to proactively focus on providing the appropriate care that chronically ill/injured patients require to improve quality of life and to decrease costs.

MEDICAL ASPECTS OF CHRONIC ILLNESS AND DISABILITY

As noted in the introduction, more than one in five adults are living with chronic conditions at a cost of $234 billion in lost productivity, and $425 billion in medical spending per year.[4] As daunting as these figures are, they become even higher when absenteeism is factored into the cost of lost productivity, resulting from workers who need time off to care for family members affected by chronic conditions or elder care issues. Chronic conditions such as low back pain, cancer, asthma, diabetes, and depression are examples of chronic conditions that can repeatedly render employees un- or underproductive for days, weeks, or months.

In addition to the physical aspect of illness, many people with chronic conditions, as well as family members who care for them, suffer from the emotional effects of their illness. To assist people to cope with chronic diseases, case managers must understand the medical and psychological aspects of chronic diseases, so that they can assist patients and families to change behaviors that will allow them to more readily adapt to their conditions, and to learn self-management skills. When patients are empowered to self manage, adherence to the plan of care increases, techniques are used to better manage complications, and disability is minimized.

The skills that patients need to self-manage chronic conditions are difficult to develop and hard to sustain. The first step case managers can take to assist the patient and family in self managing a chronic illness is to educate them about the disease, and what they can do to minimize its impact on their lives. Lifestyle changes, such as adopting more healthful eating habits for a newly diagnosed diabetic, or advising a patient to stop smoking if peripheral vascular disease is the problem, are difficult but essential to decrease complications related to their disease processes. Reinforcing what the condition is and why changes need to be made allows patients to understand how they can control disease versus having disease control them.

For case managers to be successful educators of this population, they need to have a thorough understanding of the current clinical issues pertaining to a particular disease process. Many managed care organizations offer disease management (DM) programs and have assigned case managers to specialize in particular diagnoses. Patients served by the DM program include those with high-risk pregnancies, transplants, AIDS and AIDS-related diseases, asthma, COPD, CHF, and long-term pediatric services, such as neonatal care or cancer treatment. Specialization in a specific area allows the case manager to develop relationships with providers and with centers of excellence that provide specific treatment and services. These relationships allow the case manager to meet the needs of the patient and the family more effectively and efficiently.

Managed care organizations actively identify chronic conditions that affect specific populations, and classify patients according to degree or type of risk. Those patients viewed as high risk are assigned to a case manager to effectively manage health-care services and to educate the patient/family to better self-manage their care. For example, in 1994 asthma affected an estimated 14.2 million Americans, and cost the U.S. economy an estimated $10.7 billion, according to a study sponsored by the Asthma and Allergy Foundation of America. Indirect costs of asthma in 1994 accounted for $4.64 billion in lost workdays, missed time from school and costs attributed to asthma deaths. Indirect costs went from nearly $2 billion in adjusted 1985 dollars to $4.64 billion in 1994, a 133 percent increase.[5]

Once a population is identified as having been diagnosed with asthma, a multidisciplinary team of experts constructs a proactive program to address the diverse needs of the population. These experts will work closely with the physician or nurse practitioner in charge of the patient. The physician or nurse practitioner, as the individual legally licensed to diagnose and treat a patient, is the individual most appropriate to determine the treatment plan. Managed care organizations use case managers to educate those patients most at risk, to enable them to better manage their disease. A case manager assesses patients with asthma to ensure they are using appropriate tools that allow them to maintain wellness and work toward self- management. For example, the respiratory therapist case manager monitors a patient's use of his peak flow meter. Peak flow meters allow patients with asthma to measure lung capacity and functional levels. When properly used, the meters help patients to manage activities and self-adjust medications to fit their physical and functional requirements. Readings can alert patients to conditions that require immediate medical attention, such as an upper respiratory infection that can trigger an acute episode of wheezing. Early identification allows the patient to adjust medications to control attacks. By developing a routine of regularly measuring peak flows, patients can recognize whether preventive measures are working, or if they need to seek medical attention.

Outcomes that an asthma disease management program can claim just through this singular proactive education, are:

- improved patient and provider satisfaction;
- improved clinical status;
- improved functional status;

- appropriate use of healthcare resources;
- decrease in lost time at work and school;
- decrease in healthcare spending on reactive care.

The next section addresses some of the chronic conditions that case managers proactively manage to promote health, decrease health care costs, and prevent disabilities.

PATHOPHYSIOLOGICAL CONDITIONS

Case managers are charged with managing patients with chronic conditions that result from a variety of reasons, and which span the continuum of care. To do this, case managers need to have an understanding of specific disease processes and realize how the condition, if not managed well, can impact the patient's ability to function independently. By understanding each aspect of the disease process, case managers are able to proactively manage patients and address specific needs that allow both the patient and the family to cope, to maintain a state of wellness, and to become empowered to take advantage of resources.

To be successful, case managers have the professional responsibility to stay current with advances in clinical practice. Various sources are available to case managers that provide valuable information regarding specific conditions. The Internet has a wealth of information that can be accessed in minutes from any setting. Medical texts are available resources that usually can be found in any organization's internal library. Networking and collaborating with other professionals who specialize in a specific area are helpful contacts. For example, a managed care case manager can learn the important milestones that a premature infant is expected to achieve before discharge, by consulting with a neonatal intensive care nurse. Similarly, working closely with the oncology nurse specialist gives the acute care case manager insight into specific treatments available to manage chemotherapy side effects. Recognizing and respecting the expertise of other members of the health care team allow the case manager to gain valuable expertise about patients' pathophysiologic conditions.

PSYCHOSOCIAL CONDITIONS

Chronic diseases take patients and families through periods of good health mixed with periods of sickness. During these times, patients experience a variety of emotions that can often complicate care. To support and empower patients and families to develop coping strategies, case manages are aware that each person reacts and handles problems in his/her own way. Listening to patients and family members about how they are coping is an important role that case managers play in disease management. Helping other members of the health care team to understand the challenges and stressors that affect the patient is an important function of the case manager. Being sensitive to the range of emotions that patients experience, (denial, confusion, fear, avoidance, anger, grief, and guilt) assists the case manager to see why patients act the way they do.[6]

Another aspect that confronts patients and family members dealing with chronic disease is how other people react to them because of an illness or injury that makes them "different". Support groups offer people a way to see that they are not alone, and that other people experience similar issues. Coping with a chronic illness is enhanced by how the patient was reared and taught to deal with crises. People with chronic illness find inner strength that they never knew they had. Spirituality and religion provide people with hope as they try to cope and internalize why things are happening to them.

Incorporating spirituality into the case management plan of care helps case managers to remember this important aspect. Case managers can recommend and direct patients and family members to spiritual resources that allow them to deal more effectively with a chronic illness. Another coping method is to encourage patients to keep their own treatment and side effects records to help them overcome feelings of helplessness and loss of control. Regaining control of their lives is an important step in helping patients be more compliant. The following example illustrates what can happen when people experience success through their own efforts.

John, a 50-year-old man who has just had two successive admissions for congestive heart failure, tells the managed care case manager that he is ready to commit to change the behaviors that his doctor has encouraged him to make for a long time. The case manager suggests that he record his daily weight, what he eats, the number of cigarettes he smokes in a day, and to list the times he takes his medications to see if any patterns develop. The case manager explains that this is an effective way for him to self-monitor and self-manage his response to treatment. This information will be valuable for the doctor to see at each visit.

As John makes progress, he finds that he is gaining a better understanding of his disease process and feels more control in his life. He tells the case manager that this is also a good way for him to remember what he needs to tell the doctor. He suggests to the case manager that all chronically ill patients be provided with a personal patient diary and taught how to do what he is successfully doing. The case manager passes John's recommendations to the director of the disease management program for consideration. She also captures John's observations in the file as soft outcome.

Having information gives the chronically ill or injured patient control and a purpose. Tracking the information gives the patient a way to review small gains made by adhering to the plan of care. Knowledge is power. Encouraging patients to learn about their diseases, and to discuss their course of therapy with the physician may be daunting at first. By encouraging patients to ask questions and be involved in their care plan, case managers help the patient to be a part of the team. Control though positive thinking and maintaining hope is arguably the most important trait a case manager can help patients and the families to develop and maintain. Having a positive attitude is key to fighting and winning the battle of chronic disease.

INFORMATION SYSTEMS

As demonstrated throughout this chapter, the main goal of disease management is to curtail the disease process and prevent exacerbations. Early interventions ensure proper use of health care resources. To be effective in managing health, a coordinated disease management program must be in place and linked to an information system that facilitates data collection, analysis, and reporting to show positive outcomes that support the need for the program.

Disease management information systems are very sophisticated. They allow organizations to collect demographic information on the population being served to plan appropriate networks, providers, resources, and staff expertise to manage specific diseases. Claims information is collected that provides valuable information about use of health care services. Programs are designed to track patient populations through the continuum of care, and link pharmacy and laboratory databases to determine what medications are prescribed by various providers in the plan, and diagnostic test results can be viewed as soon as they are available. Data are discussed with the pertinent physician to make timely and proactive changes in treatment plans. Alert mechanisms can be programmed to notify the case manager and provider that a lab value is abnormal, that a new medication added to the profile was never picked up by the patient, or that a setback occurred. These alerts trigger the case manager to follow up with the patient to see what happened, and to intervene as needed. If a hospitalization occurs, a review of the plan of care will be done to see why the admission occurred.

Often, a complication develops that changes the patient's overall condition and, therefore, the treatment plan. Consider John, who has been followed in the CHF program and has been doing well. One day the case manager receives a system alert that the patient was admitted. She calls the hospital, and finds out that the patient was involved in an auto accident and has a concussion; he was admitted for 24-hour observation. The case manager contacts the hospital to make sure that they are aware of the patient's history and current treatment plan. She also contacts John's family to mobilize resources for an early and uneventful discharge.

Another feature that a disease management information system offers is to incorporate applicable clinical guidelines to minimize variation in care. This detailed, organized information is available to all providers and increases their awareness of treatment guidelines appropriate for the patient, and to monitor aspects of patient care from remote locations. Intelligent software, as it is known, enables programs to combine all information collected and to print reports regarding practice patterns and responses to treatment. Coupled with variance tracking is the system's ability to track and analyze risks of necessary patient interventions, so that the organization can be aware in advance as to the services likely to be needed. Risks are identified and patients classified according to level of risk. More information on risk stratification will be discussed in the next section.

Disease management information systems allow treatment guidelines to be developed, enabling health care professionals involved with the patient to understand who can make changes to the plan of care, and when and how these changes can occur.[7] These guidelines streamline the process, avoid duplication and fragmentation, and allow patients' care to be provided in an organized and proactive manner that ensures services are appropriate and provided in the right setting, and at the right time.

RISK STRATIFICATION

For a disease management program to be successful, it is mandatory for an organization to determine what diseases or conditions need to be managed. The decision about which diseases are most critical to manage, is based on answers to the following questions:

- What conditions are commonly encountered in the population served?
- Which costs related to care are most significant?
- What are the variations in care, outcomes, and costs related to specific diseases?
- What is the evidence that supports best practices that can be incorporated into treatment plans to achieve predictable, improved, outcomes?[8]

Once diseases are diagnosed, the next step is to clearly define the population affected. An information system that incorporates resource utilization data, such as ICD-9 codes, provides information about specific diagnoses and procedures used to treat these conditions. The next step is to stratify those at risk for over-utilization of services or exacerbations of their illness, based on their level of risk. This essential step identifies interventions to be targeted to those patients most likely to benefit.

For example, some patients with CHF may be managing their condition well, while others are not as successful. Proactive management of all patients is important, but to be effective and address those most in need, resources are focused on those who are at high risk for poor management. Claims data to pinpoint use of services, such as frequency of ED visits, frequency of hospitalization, frequency of visits to the primary care physician or specialist, and prescribed high-cost medications are indicators used in risk stratification.

The use of risk stratification screening tools is another method of stratifying patients. Many non-profit organizations provide disease-specific screening tools that are helpful in stratifying patients according to severity of disease. The following are examples:

- The New York Heart Association's classification of patients with heart failure is available from the American Heart Association at www.americanheart.org
- The National Heart, Lung, and Blood Institute's classification of asthma severity is available at www.nhlbi.nih.gov
- The American College of Chest Physicians provides a Classification of Level of Risk for Deep Vein Thrombosis at www.chestnet.org

Identification of the population most appropriate for disease management is done, allowing those members of the health plan to be notified, who will explain the program to patients and families, and obtain their approval to participate in the program. This is most effectively achieved when the primary care physician or a member of the health care plan approaches the patient and family. Once permission is granted, patients receive written information about the disease management program and how it works.

The patient is told that the disease management program does not replace the primary care doctor, but is intended to assist the primary care physician to manage their condition in a more proactive manner.

INTERVENTIONS

Various interventions are used in disease management programs to meet the needs of patients. These interventions include providing individualized case management services, telemonitoring services, and direct contact with physicians. Programs use various combinations of interventions to meet specific population needs. Patients most at risk are assigned a case manager who works one-on-one with them to identify barriers to care, and to implement a plan of care best suited to patient needs. Telemonitoring is used and is most effective in remote areas for patients who are at moderate risk. Direct physician intervention occurs when physicians agree to participate in the program, and wish to manage their own patients. Family physicians develop disease management programs for their practices to improve outcomes. Other physicians who are members of health plans may selectively participate in disease management programs and perform special functions.

Integrated programs include physician management, use treatment guidelines to decrease variation in care, and allow patients most at risk to receive individual case management services, which is the first step in moving to a health care system that is truly concerned with managing both patient care and cost. The next section reviews information regarding interventions that are patient-focused, to improve health and decrease costs regarding chronic medical conditions.

Patient-Focused Interventions

Patient-focused Interventions are typically educational and behavioral programs that intervene to help patients to self-manage. Patients who are in a disease- management program receive periodic and ongoing educational materials specific to their disease. The goal is to change behaviors that reduce risk and enable the patient and/or family to self-manage more effectively. A case manager works directly with patients who are most at risk, to identify barriers and behaviors that may be causing problems. Interventions may be clinical, socio-cultural, financial, or behavioral. The case manager's primary goal is to improve health care outcomes.

For example, a patient who has diabetes and is obese is identified as having made several ED visits over the past month for treatment of hypoglycemia. The health plan's disease management case manager contacts the patient and learns that she has been trying to lose weight, eating only one meal a day. The patient states she thought she was doing a good thing, since she was still taking her insulin. The case manager explains that this is very dangerous since the dose of insulin is based on several factors, including diet. The case manager arranges a consult with a dietician case manager. The dietician case manager telephonically contacts the patient and addresses the importance of adhering to a special nutritional diet that allows the patient to gain better control of her glucose while reducing her weight. The dietitian provides a detailed meal plan to the patient and makes certain that the patient fully understands both diet and insulin dosage. She also gives the patient a list of weight reduction support programs available in the community. Two weeks later the dietician case manager follows up with the patient, who reports that she is doing well, has lost five pounds, that her blood glucose readings are close to normal at every reading, and that she is feeling much better.

This example shows that, many times, patients have good intentions, but do not understand the consequences of their actions. The disease management case manager is able to identify barriers and behaviors that may be causing problems, and then to mobilize resources to minimize use of health care resources, while maximizing quality of life for the patient. When follow-up occurs, the patient is able to report success, and her sense of worth is enhanced.

Patient-Focused Medication Compliance

Without appropriate medication compliance, even the best therapies will not work. Studies show that fifty percent of hospitalizations for CHF are preventable, and that medication noncompliance is a major reason for an exacerbation of CHF to occur.[9] Monitoring compliance is one of the interventions used to reinforce patient education and to help identify early warning signs of worsening CHF, to avoid a crisis. This is shown in the following case study.

A home care case manager was notified by the disease management case manager to work with Mr. Smith, following his third admission for shortness of breath in six weeks. The home care case manager met with Mr. Smith in his home. She noted that the home was very stuffy and asked if he had an air conditioner. Mr. Smith stated that his A/C unit broke, and he had been unable to get it fixed. She asked him to let her see his medications. Mr. Smith gave her his bottles. The case manager counted the pills and noted that there were too many pills left in the bottle of Lasix™. In discussing this with Mr. Smith, he told the case manager that he took the medication only when his feet swelled, since the medication made him wake up at least four times a night to go to the bathroom. The case manager asked Mr. Smith when he was taking the medication, and he reported taking it before going to bed. The case manager explained to him that the pills would make him urinate often, and advised him to take the medication early in the morning, on arising. She emphasized the importance of taking the Lasix™ daily as prescribed. The case manager asked Mr. Smith if he would like a pill holder. She could mark the times for him to take each medication on the holder. He was grateful to receive the pill holder. She informed him that most discount pharmacy stores carry a supply of pill holders should he need another. She advised him to keep track of his weight on a daily basis, to ensure that the medications were working. She also inquired if he had family members who could help in paying to have the A/C unit fixed. He said his son could probably help him out, but he had not asked for help because he was managing the heat OK. The home care case manager explained to Mr. Smith how the increased heat was requiring his body to work harder to stay cool, placing increased effort on his heart. Knowing this, Mr. Smith agreed to contact his son for help. The home care case manager followed up with Mr. Smith one week later. He was doing better. He was taking his medications as she had directed, and had lost 7 pounds. His legs were not swollen, and he was able to get around the house without tiring so easily. His son sent a handyman over to fix the air conditioner so that now he was able to stay cool, which he noticed was really helping his breathing.

This case study illustrates that medication noncompliance can be caused by factors other than just not taking the medication. In this situation, the noncompliance was due to lack of education about how to take medication at the appropriate time. Although Mr. Smith may have been informed by the physician regarding when and how to take Lasix™, he may have been too overwhelmed or too weak at the time to concentrate on the instructions, and did not read the written information provided by the pharmacy when his prescription was filled. Periodically reinforcing education about compliance with medication helps the patient to appropriately adhere to the treatment plan. Exploring reasons why a patient is noncompliant may elicit situations that might never be discussed by the patient with his/her primary care physician, but which could affect treatment significantly.

Patient-Focused Behavior Modification

One of the goals of an effective disease management program is preventing disease for those at risk. An example illustrating that behavior modification is essential to achieve long-term prevention is that of weight management. Obesity is now at epidemic levels across all age groups.[10] Adults have many resources, but for young children and adolescents, resources are either not available or not suitable. Childhood obesity is a serious and growing problem that is predictive of medical complications and higher costs later in life. Weight reduction programs designed for children are geared to boost self-esteem, communication skills, and self-confidence while promoting healthy eating habits.[11] Pediatric behavior modification programs focus more on a conservative, multidisciplinary approach that does not emphasize dieting. The key to a successful pediatric obesity management program is educating both the parents and the children about the importance of good nutrition, exercise, and being able to take responsibility for one's behavior. Proactively encouraging behavior modification early helps children to successfully acquire knowledge and to develop abilities that last a lifetime.

Patient-Focused Disease Monitoring

To manage chronic illness/injury proactively, patients must be aware of early, subtle changes in the their condition. Those who work closely with patients teach them to report any changes to their physicians. If a pattern is evident, the physician or case manager attempts to identify the problem so that adjustments can be made. Unfortunately, some patients are reluctant to contact their doctors or feel that if they do report problems often they will be seen as problem patients. Disease management programs try to dispel this feeling, and encourage patients to report even normal information to providers so that the team can include positive information as well as negative information in outcomes reports. This proactive approach is essential for disease management programs to work effectively, and to allow providers to learn more about disease progression.

In a sense, disease monitoring allows each disease management program to be its own research project. By gathering specific data about pertinent elements in managing specific diseases, providers gain better insight into the disease process, and can develop appropriate new interventions to more effectively manage the disease. Active participation allows patients to be more responsible for improving their disease.

Information technology enhances research efficiency by enabling patients with specific conditions, such as chronic kidney disease, to gather daily diagnostic information through the Internet, and transmit it to the physician or clinician. Patients are instructed to take their own pulse, blood pressure, weight, and to answer simple questions, such as how they are feeling, whether their feet are swollen, and whether they took their medication(s) as instructed. When patients enter this information into a telemonitoring device, it is transmitted to a central office where the information is entered into a computer, analyzed, and made available to the clinicians participating in the disease management program. Red flags are programmed into the computer to alert providers about blood pressure that is too high or too low, or weight gain or loss This information is used to determine whether medications need to be changed, or whether the patient requires further evaluation.

Patient-Focused Disease Prevention

The primary goals of disease prevention are to prolong life, to decrease morbidity, and to improve quality of life. Incorporating disease management principles into the health care system enables health care professionals to analyze information about patients' personal health and family history, health behaviors, and environmental and cultural issues that result in the development of chronic disease or catastrophic events, such as a heart attack or stroke. This technology is still in its beginning stages, but health care organizations continue to focus on the ability to provide the current data that can improve patient care.[12]

In addition to tools that predict risk, a mind shift is needed regarding how the general public perceives health and wellness. Educational efforts that support changes in behaviors need to be incorporated into the mainstream so that the public can "get the message". An example of how one state was able to influence change and prevent disease is seen in a report showing the effects of California's tough antismoking laws. Evidence proves that lung cancer is directly related to smoking. Lung cancer incidence in California began dropping in the late 1980s, helped partly by Proposition 99, a law to ban smoking in public places. State health care officials reported the results of a ten-year study showing a 14% decrease in lung cancer in California. The Center for Disease Control and Prevention (CDC) reports that other regions of the country reported only a 2.7% decrease over the same period.[13] Case managers and health care providers should be active in their individual states to emphasize efforts to reduce risk behaviors that will result in prevention of disease at the consumer level.

Provider-Focused Interventions

As health care providers, our satisfaction at the end of the day comes from knowing that we were able to provide quality care to patients. Case managers and primary care physicians, working together in a primary health care practice, can change behaviors of people. For these efforts to be successful, individual providers know that information about scientific advances and new drugs that are effective in treating chronic diseases, must be accessed, analyzed, and incorporated into practice.

Considering the speed at which new treatment information is growing, and the pace of change in the current health care climate, keeping up with new information is a challenge that all health care professionals struggle to meet. To streamline this process, individual providers as well as large organizations are implementing several types of data management systems to rapidly disseminate new information. A data systems approach allows providers and health care professionals to focus on particular disease processes, include evidence-based treatment guidelines into their practices, and implement programs that identifies those at risk earlier. This approach improves the quality of health care and allows resources to be allocated efficiently and effectively. Information on data management systems was covered in Chapter four.

Provider-Focused Treatment Guidelines

Treatment guidelines are tools designed to help practitioners and patients make decisions about appropriate health care for specific conditions, and which are vital to the success of any disease management program. The major objective is to use guidelines that are evidence-based, disease-specific and user-friendly. Collaborating with those providers who use guidelines is essential for positive patient outcomes. Choosing physicians who encourage/persuade other physicians and providers to use treatment guidelines is important in deciding who will be members of the multidisciplinary team active in developing specific guidelines.

Treatment guidelines are intended to improve care for a specifically targeted disease management population by decreasing variation in care of specific conditions. The cornerstone of treatment guidelines is that they are based on scientific, accepted, consistent practice in the health care community. Once developed, guidelines can be applied to patients who present with a specific condition, and used to monitor the effectiveness of interventions. Outcomes generated from treatment protocols should support best practices. As the term treatment guidelines suggests, they are used to guide care. Every physician and healthcare professional is expected to use independent clinical judgment when caring for patients, since response to treatment can vary from patient to patient. Additional information on treatment guidelines is addressed in Chapter four.

Provider-Focused Behavior Modification

Of the more than two million deaths occurring in the U.S. each year, as many as 50% may be due to preventable causes. Lifestyle and behavior play a central role in the cause of morbidity and mortality.[14] Helping patients to change behavior to improve health, and to prevent catastrophic events and chronic disease is an important role for the disease management case manager. Interventions that promote behavior change are in modifying lifestyle to prevent disease, manage long-term disease management, and improve quality of life. Understanding a patient's readiness to make changes, identifying and appreciating barriers to change, and helping patients anticipate setbacks can improve patient satisfaction and reduce frustration among health care members.

Understanding the stages of change experienced by those with chronic illness is necessary for health care professionals to design behavior modification programs. Change in behavior occurs gradually, with the patient moving from being uninterested, unaware, or unwilling to make a change, to considering a change, to deciding and preparing to make a change. At this stage, determined action is taken and, the new behavior continues over time until it becomes habitual. Setbacks are common, and must become part of the process of working toward life-long change.[15]

PHARMACOECONOMICS

The last section in this chapter provides information on pharmaco-economics as a part of any successful disease management program. Pharmaco-economics is a branch of economics that applies cost-benefit, cost-effectiveness, cost-minimization, and cost-utility analyses in comparing the economics of different pharmaceutical products and drug therapies.[16] This information is helpful as pharmaceutical companies factor in these data to base decisions about producing new drugs, or continuing to produce older drugs.

As more expensive drugs become available, questions and concerns are raised by payers, government officials, health care professionals, and the public regarding the cost versus the effectiveness of drugs. Pharmaco-economic data become important in making informed decisions about drugs placed on formularies. Formularies are lists of drugs approved for use in various sectors of the healthcare system. For example, the formulary of an HMO will include certain trade drugs and certain generic drugs approved by the HMO for payment. The formulary system is used by hospitals, managed care organizations, Medicare, Medicaid, and insurance companies.

The goal of a formulary in any disease management program is to guide rational drug use efficiently, control costs, and improve delivery of health care services for patients with a specific disease process. Formulary prices are negotiated, since disease management programs offer high-volume use of drug products for targeted populations. Formulary policies and clinical practice guidelines have a significant impact on the prescribing practices of many physicians, who are forced to change prescribing behaviors to comply with the disease management formulary.

REFERENCES

1. Prochaska, J. Helping cure healthcare systems: changing minds and behavior. *Disease Management Outcomes*. 1999: 6,6:335–341.
2. National Center for Chronic Disease Prevention and Health Promotion. *About chronic disease*. Available at: www.cdc.gov/nccdphp/about.htm
3, 9. James, M. At the heart of the disease management revolution. *The Case Manager*. 1998: 7:47–50.
4. Patients as effective collaborators in managing chronic conditions. Available at: http://www.milbank.org/990811chronic.html
5. Asthma and Allergy Foundation of America website. http://www.aafa.org/templ/display.cfm?id=16&sub=67. Accessed 12.16.04
6. National Institute of Health. Coping with chronic illness. *Patient Information Publications*. Bethesda, MD. Warren Grant Magnuson Clinical Center. 1996; 1–10.
7. Kibbe, D, Johnson, K. Do-it-yourself disease management. *Family Practice Management*. 1998: 36,11:1–10.
8. Rivo, M. It's time to start practicing population-based health care. *Family Practice Management*. 1998: 8,6:63–76.
10, 11. Faler, C, Levick, K. Pioneering programs making a dent in childhood obesity. *Disease Management Advisor*. 2000: 6,8:123–127.
13. Coleman, J. CDC lung cancer: anti-tobacco measures lessen cancer. Available at: http://www.cdc.gov/mmwr/preview/mmwrhtml/ mm4947a4.htm
14, 15. Zimmerman, G, Olsen, C. Stages of change- approach to helping patients change behavior. American Family Physician. 2000: 3,1:1–12.
16. University of Dundee. Pharmacoeconomics: a brief history. Available at: http://www.dundee.ac.uk/memo/memoonly/PHECO0.HTM

HEALTH CARE LEGISLATION

8

For several years, U.S.-based case managers have been pursuing case management certification, meeting demanding eligibility criteria for national examinations. They report that one of the most surprising aspects of these examinations is the focus on legislation. There is reason to require that case managers in all practice settings possess sufficient understanding of health care legislation as part of the case management core body of knowledge. Health care legislation impacts cost, quality, and access to health care in this country. Health care legislation impacts *who* will achieve access to health care, *what* health care benefits will be accessed, *where* health care will be accessed or denied, *why* health care is delivered in the manner it is within the systems and processes, *how* health care is delivered, and *when* health care systems and benefits can be accessed by various populations.

In addition to understanding how health care legislation affects health care delivery for the patients/families served, case managers must continuously monitor whether their practice is consistent with current legislation. This involves having knowledge of pertinent legislation at the local, state and federal levels. This chapter provides a useful resource and review guide to assist the case manager in obtaining a working knowledge of federal legislation affecting rehabilitation, managed care, disability, and employment settings. Case managers must be cautioned that our democracy provides for the continual and potential impact of new or changing health care legislation, so that this chapter will never be complete. As consumers become more demanding of patient-centered care and patient rights, changes in health care delivery will be reflected in local, state, and federal legislation mandates. Further, case managers as advocates have a responsibility to become involved in legislation that will enhance health care quality, cost and access for all consumers. Therefore, case managers should commit to an ongoing study of—and a participation in—the dynamic health care legislative process.

Case managers can participate in, and gain current knowledge of health care policy through professional organizations, such as the American Nurses Association (ANA), or the Case Management Society of America (CMSA). They can contact their local legislators and request to be added to mailing lists to receive any free consumer-based legislative updates or newsletters. They can seek valid, accurate data from the Federal Register or other published government monographs. These are available through local libraries, the law libraries of any university, and online at various websites, such as www.firstgov.gov, or www.whitehouse. gov. However, case managers should always check sources carefully, particularly when accessing information from the Internet.

The following legislation is basic in influencing patients and providers associated with case management practice.

REHABILITATION LEGISLATION
Rehabilitation Act of 1973

Section 501: This section of the Act promulgates basic federal law containing programs and civil rights for all persons with disabilities.

Section 502: This section is an amendment to the Rehabilitation Act enacted in 1978. It pertains to the governance and accessibility laws provided by the Architectural and Transportation Barriers Compliance Board (ATBCB).

Section 503: This is an amendment to the Rehabilitation Act pertaining to affirmative action for persons with disabilities. Compliance is required by federal employers, or by entities operating in federal locations, or funded with federal dollars.

Section 504: This amendment to the Rehabilitation Act pertains to non-discrimination of persons with disabilities by the federal government or by entities operating in federal locations, or funded with federal dollars.

Social Security Act of 1935

This Act established vocational rehabilitation as a permanent federal program in 1935. When individuals apply under any one of the disability provisions of the Social Security law, they are automatically referred to individual state vocational rehabilitation programs. Agencies and eligibility for services vary state to state; however, states are responsible for providing counseling, training, and/or other services to support the return of disabled individuals to work on a part-time or full-time basis.

Smith-Hughes Act of 1917

This legislation provides matching federal funds to states for vocational education programs that were implemented prior to enactment of permanent programs through the Social Security Act.

Smith-Fess Act of 1920

Also known as the Civilian Vocational Rehabilitation Act, this legislation provides for the initiation of civilian vocational rehabilitation programs.

MANAGED CARE LEGISLATION
Emergency Medical Treatment and Active Labor Act (EMTALA)

Passed in 1986, this Act applies to all hospitals receiving Medicare funds and maintaining an emergency room. Also known as the "patient dumping law", this Act requires emergency rooms to screen a patient to determine whether the patient suffers from an emergency medical condition or if a pregnant patient is in active labor, before asking the patient about ability to pay or method of payment. If the patient is found to be suffering from an emergency medical condition or is in active labor, the hospital must provide necessary and appropriate treatment to stabilize the patient. The hospital cannot delay treatment to determine payer benefits. In amendments to the law passed in 1989, specialty hospitals (ie, burn unit, trauma center) must accept transfer of a patient requiring special treatment available at the facility. The Act also prevents hospitals from admitting the patient and then immediately discharging the patient in an effort to circumvent the law.

EMTALA also governs a managed care company's request to have a patient transferred from a non-participating hospital in the managed care network, to a participating hospital in the managed care network. Before the request can be fulfilled, the acute care-based case manager will need to ensure that the patient is medically stable for transfer; that the treating physician authorizes transfer; that there is a treating physician willing to accept the patient at the new facility; that the patient has consented to the transfer; and that the patient's medical records accompany the patient at the time of transfer.

Health Insurance Portability and Accountability Act (HIPAA) of 1996

There are several components to this comprehensive legislative Act.

- Limits the exclusion period for pre-existing conditions mandated by insurance companies to 12 months;

- Allows employees to be automatically eligible for benefits without pre-existing conditions when assuming new employment, providing there has not been a break in the employee's group coverage for more than 62 days;
- Provides for a tax-qualified long-term care benefit;
- Allows Medical Savings Accounts (MSA) on a trial basis for employers with under 50 employees;
- Provides establishment of the Patient Privacy Regulations, which were released by the Health and Human Services (HHS) Department on December 20, 2000, and governs the confidentiality of medical records, including electronic records, printouts of such records, paper records, and even oral communications.

The HIPAA Privacy Rule

The Standards for Privacy of Individually Identifiable Health Information (Privacy Rule) establishes a national set of standards for the protection of certain health information. The U.S. Department of Health and Human Services (HHS) issues the Privacy Rule under the Health Insurance Portability and Accountability Act of 1996. The Privacy Rule is intended to protect the use and disclosure of individuals' health information, known as protected health information (PHI) by organizations subject to the Privacy Rule. With the HHS, the Office for Civil Rights (OCR) has responsibility to implement and enforce the Privacy Rule with respect to voluntary compliance activities and civil money penalties.

One of the major objectives of the Privacy Rule is to protect individuals' health information while, at the same time, allowing the flow of health information required to provide and promote quality health care and to protect the public's health and well being. Because of the diversity of the health care industry, the Privacy Rule is designed to be flexible and comprehensive to cover a variety of circumstances and disclosures that need to be addressed.[1]

Under the Patient Privacy Regulations of HIPAA, health care providers and systems are required to implement policies and procedures to uphold the privacy and exchange of PHI data. They are also responsible to train every existing and new workplace employee and member on their respective HIPAA privacy policies and procedures. This requirement became effective April 14, 2003, and essentially requires every employee to minimally know the following:

1. What HIPAA is
2. Who the entity's HIPAA Privacy Official is
3. What are the entity's protected health information (PHI) limits pertaining to patients (what is each employee's level of access to PHI information)
4. Where to obtain a copy of the entity's Privacy Notice
5. What to do when a privacy violation is witnessed
6. Knowledge that the care of the patient always takes precedence

Entities and individuals required to comply with the Privacy Rule include but are not limited to health care professionals, pharmacies, hospitals, clinics, home health care agencies, durable medical equipment companies, nursing homes, health plans, managed care organizations, employer groups and even certain government programs that pay for health care, such as Medicare and Medicaid.

Under the provisions of the Privacy Rule, individuals have the right to:
- obtain a copy of their health records
- have corrections added to their health information
- receive notices explaining how health information will be used and shared
- determine whether to give permission before private health information is used or shared for certain purposes, such as for marketing

- obtain a report on when and why health information was shared for certain purposes
- file a complaint with a provider or health insurer or the U.S. Government if there is cause to believe that rights are being denied or health information is not being protected

Omnibus Budget Reconciliation Act (OBRA) 1989, 1990

OBRA is a broad-based legislative Act with many implications. In these 1989 and 1990 amendments of the OBRA Act, individual states are required to provide Medicaid coverage for all pregnant women and their children up to six years of age if the family income is less than 133% of the federal poverty level. Also formed from this Act was the Agency for Health Care Policy and Research,* which continues to be an active overseer of managed care and health care delivery.

Patient Self-Determination Act of 1990

Written in 1990 and enacted in 1991, the Patient Self-Determination Act requires that health care facilities in the U.S. advise patients upon admission of their right to accept or refuse treatment should they become gravely ill. The following facilities must comply with the law: hospitals, hospice, sub-acute, skilled nursing facilities, and home health care agencies that accept Medicaid or Medicare patients. Under the Act, patients are entitled to advance directives (living wills and Durable Power of Attorney proxies). *Living wills* designate whether an individual desires life-prolonging treatment in the event s/he is unable to make medical decisions. A *Durable Power of Attorney* designates who will make health care decisions in the event s/he is unable to make medical decisions.

The Act requires health care providers to perform the following:

- Provide adult patients with written notification of their state law regarding the right to refuse treatment and advance directives; and provide the policies of the facility or agency;
- Document in the patient's medical record whether he/she has advance directives;
- Ensure compliance with applicable state laws on advance directives;
- Create and maintain policies and procedures on advance directives, and educate the staff regarding these policies and procedures.

A facility or health care provider cannot require patients to execute advance directives as a condition of treatment or admission.[2]

Uniform Anatomical Gifts Act

All hospitals receiving Medicare or Medicaid funding are required to establish written guidelines for identifying potential organ donors under the Uniform Anatomical Gifts Act. A potential donor is defined as a person who dies in circumstances that are generally acceptable for donation of at least one solid organ if the donor can be identified in a timely manner, and if permission for the donation is obtained.

DISABILITY LEGISLATION
Americans with Disabilities Act of 1990

This has been the most comprehensive, complex legislation passed to date to protect the rights of disabled individuals. Broad legislation is defined through five distinct sections, known as Titles.

Title I: Pertains to employment provisions and has been enforced by the Equal Employment Opportunity Commission (EEOC), Washington, D.C., since July 26, 1992. Effective July 26, 1994, companies with 15 or more employees must comply with the mandates of Title 1. *See Employer Section of this chapter for further information.*

---

*This agency is now known as the Agency for Health Care Research and Quality

Title II: Pertains to public transportation, providing for access to public transportation by all disabled individuals. Enforcement is by the Department of Transportation (DOT), Washington, D.C. Examples of mandated provisions include: wheelchair lifts included on public transportation (city buses), and on private transportation accessed by the public (car rental shuttle buses).

Title III: Pertains to public access provisions, providing for accessible public accommodations in all settings visited or used by disabled citizens. Title III has been federally enforced since January 1, 1993, by the Department of Justice (DOJ) in Washington, D.C.

Title IV: Pertains to accessible transmitting and telecommunication devices (TDDs). Affects telecommunications companies and all industries using these devices (ie, hotel telephones, hospital television sets)

Title V: Pertains to arbitration, and allows a legal process by which a disabled individual can seek restitution.

Architectural Barriers Act of 1968

This Act requires federal and federally assisted buildings and facilities to be accessible to, and usable by, persons with disabilities.

Education for All Handicapped Children Act (EAHCA)

This legislation provides the right to all disabled children to receive "free appropriate public education" and extensive "due process" procedures. The Act promotes equal educational opportunities despite the child's degree of disability or services needed to achieve equality. It establishes procedures by which disabled children are evaluated and their classifications determined. It then provides for the development and implementation of appropriate programs of special education and "related services" stemming from the evaluations and classifications. These are known as Individualized Education Programs (IEP) and must be developed jointly by school officials and parents.[3]

Social Security Disability Income (SSDI)

SSDI legislation provides for disability insurance, as part of the federal social security program, to replace part of earnings lost because of any physical or mental impairment severe enough to prevent an individual from working. Monthly case benefits are paid to eligible disabled persons and to eligible auxiliary beneficiaries (ie, eligible person's minor children) throughout a period of disability after an initial five-month waiting period.

Social Security Act of 1935

The Social Security Act established vocational rehabilitation as a permanent federal program in 1935.

Urban Mass Transit Act

The Act provides special provisions for handicapped and elderly people in public transportation, and stood alone as a transportation related access law until the A.D.A. was enacted.

EMPLOYER LEGISLATION
Title I of the Americans with Disabilities Act (ADA)

Title I of the ADA pertains to employment provisions and has been enforced by the Equal Employment Opportunity Commission (EEOC) in Washington, D.C., since July 26, 1992. Effective July 26, 1994, companies with 15 or more employees were required to comply with the mandates of Title I. Employers may not discriminate against qualified individuals seeking a job offer or holding a job. Employers must reasonably accommodate the disabilities of qualified applicants or employees, including modifying work stations and equipment, unless an undue hardship to the company would result. Undue hardship is determined on a case-by-case basis by the EEOC and/or through the arbitration process under Title

V of the Act. Individuals may file complaints with the EEOC, or via a private lawsuit after exhausting administrative remedies. Remedies are the same as those available under Title VII of the Civil Rights Act of 1964. The court may order the employer to hire or promote qualified individuals, reasonably accommodate their disabilities, and/or pay back wages and attorneys' fees.

FACTS TO KNOW UNDER TITLE I OF THE ADA
Essential Job Function

If a person is otherwise qualified to perform a job description, but cannot perform one or more essential job functions due to disability, reasonable accommodation must be made for the disabled employee. Essential job functions are defined by the employer. It is the responsibility of the employer to have written job descriptions, and to state all of the essential job functions in each written job description.

- The function must be highly specialized.
- Existing employees performing the job description must be required to perform the function noted as an essential job function.
- Removing the essential job function must fundamentally change the job.
- There must be a limited number of employees able to perform the function or among whom the function can be distributed.

Reasonable Accommodation and Undue Hardship

A reasonable accommodation is defined as any change in the work environment or in the way things are usually done that results in equal employment opportunity for an individual with a disability.[4] Employers are obligated to make reasonable accommodation unless they can show that the accommodation would cause an undue hardship on the operation of the business. Undue hardship is defined as excessively costly, extensive, substantial, or disruptive, or that would fundamentally alter the nature or operation of the business.[5]

An example of reasonable accommodation: A disabled employee must have equal access to lunchrooms, employee lounges, restrooms, meeting rooms, and any employer sponsored services, such as health programs, transportation, and social events.

Consolidated Omnibus Budget Reconciliation Act (COBRA)

This Act passed in 1986 requires employers and their health insurance group plans to provide temporary extension of health benefits coverage to an employee, the spouse and any dependent children after the employee leaves a job. Coverage must be offered for a fixed period of time at a predetermined group rate. The employee must be covered under the employer's group health insurance plan in order to qualify, even if the employee is only covered for one day at the time of departure from the job. Employers are also required to offer COBRA benefits to divorced or widowed spouses of employees, and former dependent children of employees under the Act.

The following scenarios qualify as "leaving the job":

- Voluntary resignation
- Strike or walk-out
- Lay-off or reduction in hours
- Termination (not through gross misconduct)
- Death
- Retirement
- Entitlement of the employee to Medicare coverage
- Dependent child's loss of dependence by reaching a certain age

COBRA benefits are available to employees and family members for 18 months. However, if spouses and dependents of an employee have coverage as a result of the employee's death, divorce, legal separation, age limitation, or the employee's eligibility for Medicare, spouses and dependents are entitled to 36 months of coverage.

ERISA

The Employment Retirement Income Security Act (ERISA) of 1974 sets minimum standards for pension plans in private industry. ERISA applies two types of private employee benefit plans—pension plans and employee welfare benefit plans, which provide benefits in the event of sickness, hospitalizations, surgery, accident, death, disability or unemployment. Of note is that ERISA exempts nongovernmental, self-insured employee benefit plans from meeting the minimum benefit regulations required of other nongovernmental insurance companies.

Fair Labor Standards Act

This Act serves as the cornerstone of federal worker protection. It provides a minimum hourly wage, requires payment of additional compensation for overtime, regulates child labor, and prohibits working from home in certain industries. The Fair Labor Standards Act is enforced by the U.S. Department of Labor's Wage-Hour Division.

Family and Medical Leave Act of 1993 (FMLA)

The FMLA requires covered employers to provide up to 12 weeks of unpaid, job protected leave in a 12-month period to eligible employees for certain family and medical reasons. Employees are eligible if they have worked for a covered employer for at least one year, and for 1,250 hours over the previous 12 months. The employer is eligible if there are at least 50 employees employed within 75 miles. During the leave, the employer must maintain health benefits for the employee if the employee desires. However, the employer is not required to pay health benefits beyond the 12 weeks if the employee cannot return to work. In this scenario, COBRA benefits would be assigned (see COBRA under the Managed Care section of this chapter). Employees are entitled to work fewer hours per week or per work day if the serious health condition warrants reduction in work time. The employer is entitled to require that the serious health condition be certified by a health care provider.

Unpaid leave must be granted for any of the following reasons:

- to care for the employee's child after birth, or placement for adoption or foster care;
- to care for the employee's spouse, son or daughter, or parent who has a serious health problem;
- to attend to a serious health condition that makes the employee unable to perform his/her job.

At the employer or employee discretion, certain kinds of paid leave may be substituted for unpaid leave. These may include short- or long-term disability benefits. The FMLA is enforced by the U.S. Department of Labor, which is authorized to investigate and resolve complaints of violations by the employee or by the employer.

Longshore and Harbor Workers' Compensation Act of 1928

First enacted in 1928, with amendments in 1972 to broaden those covered under the Act, this Act is administered by the Department of Labor through the Office of Workers' Compensation. It provides medical and financial benefits to longshoremen and harbor workers while they are unable to work, including job modifications and retraining when the worker is able to resume work. The claims examiner acts as a case manager responsible for the financial and medical direction of the case, and refers the client to a rehabilitation specialist. Vocational rehabilitation is not mandatory under the Act.

Occupational Safety and Health Administration Act (OSHA)

The OSHA Act establishes OSHA as the primary regulatory system for workplace health and safety. OSHA rules include numerous safety standards and requirements for employers. It also requires employers to maintain injury records and provide employees with information about hazards in the workplace. States are free to establish their own OSHA agencies, provided the safety requirements are at least as stringent as those at the federal level.

Omnibus Budget Reconciliation Act (OBRA) of 1986

In another move to make Medicare the secondary payer behind employer group health benefit plans (see TEFRA below), this Act mandates that employer plans are first payer for employees or their dependents who are permanently disabled and Medicare-eligible. As stated earlier in this chapter, OBRA is a broad-based legislative Act with many implications. This chapter offers brief encapsulations of specific components of legislation.

Tax Equity and Fiscal Responsibility Act (TEFRA) of 1982

This Act amended the Social Security Act, making Medicare the secondary payer behind employer group health benefit plans for employees and their spouses between the ages of 65–69. Under the Act, employers are required to offer employees aged 65–69 the same health benefits as those offered to younger employees. Then in 1986, the employer's plan became the primary payer for ALL active, Medicare-eligible employees and their spouses, regardless of age.

Workers' Compensation Act of 1911

This Act established a no-fault system that provided workers' compensation laws in 10 states originally. It requires the employer to assume the cost of occupational disability, death or disease without regard to fault. All state workers' compensation systems provide wage replacement for both temporary and permanent disabilities, regardless of whether the employer or the worker is at fault for the injury or illness.

Case Managers must maintain contemporary knowledge of the legislation impacting their practice with patients or providers. New legislation and amendments to existing legislation are examples of policy mandates influencing practice.

REFERENCES

1. Summary of the HIPAA Privacy Rule. U.S. Department of Health and Human Services Website. <www.hhs.gov/ocr/privacysummary.pdf.> Accessed 12.16.04

2, 3. Romano, J. Legal rights of the catastrophically ill and injured: a family guide. Philadelphia, PA. Rosenstein & Romano,P.C. 1996:45–47.

4, 5. Americans With Disabilities Act. *Federal Register.* Washington, D.C. U.S. Government Printing Office. 1992:56,144.

REIMBURSEMENT SYSTEMS

9

Health care payer systems in the U.S. are arguably among the most diverse and complex in the world. This chapter is intended to briefly define the commonalities and differences among common reimbursement systems, and to discuss the key points necessary for a case manager to understand when navigating various payer systems. It is not intended to provide current options available in managed care plans, since benefit plans are widely variable and continue to shift to meeting the dynamic needs of the health care industry. As part of the case management process of assessment, case managers determine available benefits for a patient/family, for services and products to be provided. This requires the case manager to have a working knowledge of various reimbursement systems so that opportunities and available options can be analyzed and explored.

It is also important to realize that wide variation exists among similar reimbursement systems. For example, two patients with group health insurance benefits through their different employers may both have health maintenance organization (HMO) plans through the same insurance company. However, one plan may include a $25 co-pay for physician visits, no prescription card benefit, a limited rehabilitation benefit of 60 days, and no benefits for home health care. The other plan may offer a $10 co-pay for physician visits, a prescription card benefit that includes a $7 co-pay for brand drugs and no co-pay for generic drugs, and a 120-day benefit each for rehabilitation and home health care.

Differences are based upon the benefits menu established between each employee's company and the insurance company at the time the insurance contracts were negotiated. These differences can be confusing for provider- based case managers who may be working with several different patients and many different benefit plans, but with the same insurance company. These differences are even confusing for the case managers who work within the insurance company. They are dealing not only with different benefit plans, but are dealing with exceptions to benefits, approvals for out-of-network providers, reconsiderations, and appeals within each type of benefit plan.

Variations in health plan benefits can also be based upon whether a company offers benefit choices to its employees. Known as a cafeteria plan, different benefit choices are often provided to employees, with each employee paying different premium portions based upon the cafeteria plan selected. One employee may choose the optional dental benefits and optional long-term care benefits, while another employee may choose a lower co-payment and no prescription card benefit.

These are just a few of the examples of how health payer systems in the U.S. are among the most diverse and complex in the world. Individuals also carry private insurance because no insurance is offered through their small employers, or they may have no availability of insurance coverage through their small employer. If they have private insurance, plans can vary from managed care plans, such as HMO and PPO, to traditional indemnity plans, where there is no network of providers and much greater financial risk. Likewise, Medicare patients may have traditional indemnity Part B coverage, managed care Part B coverage, or no Part B benefits to accompany their federally funded Part A coverage. Many seniors carry special rider policies to supplement their coverage. Medicaid plans vary state to state, so that the hospital case manager may be negotiating discharge planning for two Medicaid patients with vastly different post-acute benefits and available resources. The system is no easier for the insurance-based case manager, who is expected to possess intimate knowledge of the differences in available benefits offered by his/her employer to various members in various plans.

The huge variation in reimbursement systems is further convoluted by health care legislation impacting the types of benefits offered (see Chapter eight), as well as by transition systems that shift responsibility for coverage from one reimbursement system to another. An example of this is subrogation.

SUBROGATION

Subrogation refers to the right of an insurance company or self-insured employer to be repaid for the cost of medical care or wage loss benefits. Repayment can be sought from any money a policy holder receives in a law suit or any settlement from a third party. There are many instances and many reimbursement systems in which subrogation can occur.

In workers' compensation, for example, the workers' compensation insurance company could recover a portion of medical payments and wage losses paid to an injured worker if the injured worker receives a settlement from the manufacturer of a piece of equipment that caused the injury to the worker. A similar situation could occur in health insurance, whereby medical payments are made for a policy holder injured in a skiing accident. The ski resort is later found to be negligent in allowing hazardous skiing conditions, and is required to pay a settlement. The health insurance company has a right to reimbursement from the settlement for all medical expenses paid on the skier's behalf. Likewise, an auto insurance company providing medical payments for a driver injured in a car accident can receive subrogation reimbursement from the general liability policy of the car's tire manufacturer, if defective tires on the injured driver's car are determined to have caused the auto accident.

COORDINATION OF BENEFITS

Rules exist to govern insurance plans when there are two or more types of coverage on a claim, such as when a husband and wife each have coverage for themselves and their family through employer plans, or when an employee with Medicare is still working and covered under employee health benefits. The *birthday rule* governs how to process a claim for a child who is covered under both parents' policies. The parent with the earlier birthday in the calendar year—not the older parent—is the primary benefit provider. In other words, if the father's birthday is in February and the mother's in July, the father's plan will be primary for claims processing.

A working 65-year-old woman may have both Medicare coverage and employee health benefits through her employer. In this case, health benefits will first be paid through the employer plan, and Medicare becomes a secondary payer. Further, if the woman's husband is also covered by the employer's insurance plan and by Medicare, his wife's health plan also remains primary for his health claims, with Medicare secondary.

REINSURANCE (STOP LOSS)

Another type of transition system affecting variation in reimbursement systems is reinsurance. In essence, reinsurance prevents an insurance company from going bankrupt if a large loss occurs. The term reinsurance pertains to the insuring, by one insurer, the liability of another insurer when a certain threshold has been met. This is known as a stop-loss; thus, reinsurance carriers are also known as stop-loss carriers. For example, when a group health insurance company exceeds claims of $200,000 for a plan member, the company's reinsurance company may assume the risk for any ongoing claims for that particular claim. This doesn't mean that the health insurance company is waived of its responsibility to provide coverage for the member—the member could have benefits that exceed a million dollars. What it means is that the health insurance plan's reinsurance company will reimburse claims dollars spent beyond the first $200,000.

Reinsurance coverage is common in high-risk claims, such as workers' compensation catastrophic injuries, or some high-chronicity illnesses. The re-insurer works closely with the primary insurance company, requiring notification when claims reach a certain threshold. Often the re-insurer requires that case management and utilization management be automatically assigned on or before the threshold is met as part of its stop-loss plan.

Obviously, there are countless ways in which reimbursement systems operate. Having a basic understanding of reimbursement systems will assist the case manager to know what initial questions to ask and what initial information to seek when working with a covered patient. Regardless of where the case manager practices, understanding reimbursement systems and who the key players are, assists the case manager to navigate the health care system in the best interests of the patient. This knowledge base will also continue to be both a challenge and a necessity for appropriate care coordination and intervention.

DISABILITY INSURANCE

Disability insurance generally provides periodic payments to replace income lost when an insured person is unable to work as a result of an injury or illness. Typically, disability insurance is packaged under short-term disability (STD) and long-term disability (LTD) policies that may or may not provide medical services along with wage-replacement. STD pays benefits during the time a disability exists to a covered person who remains disabled for a specified period, often not to exceed two years. LTD insurance can be issued to a group or individual to provide a reasonable replacement of a portion of income lost due to a serious or prolonged illness. STD plans can dovetail into LTD plans, or stand alone. Likewise, LTD plans can be available without STD benefits.

An important aspect of disability insurance is the "own occ/any occ" rule. Salary replacement can be based upon the plan holder's own occupation (own occ) or any comparable occupation (any occ), depending upon the plan's benefit. Under the "own occ" provision, a person may receive wage loss replacement even if limited from performing only one aspect of an entire job.

For example, an insurance-based case manager may have a chronic back injury that prevents him from driving over an extended period of time. His job as a field case manager requires him to visit hospitals all over the region once a week to review progress of members who are hospitalized. The remainder of the time, the case manager works telephonically from the insurance company's corporate office. The case manager is able to perform all other aspects of his job from his modified work station in the corporate office, even though he cannot perform the extensive traveling one day a week. Since he holds an "own occ" LTD policy, the case manager qualifies for salary replacement benefits, even though he can perform the majority of his work load.

Some plans will pay only wage losses for the policy holder's own occupation for a specific period of time; thereafter, the wage loss payments can be based upon an "any occ" rate. "Any occ" plans usually have time limitations, often being no less than one year but no more than five years. Under an "any occ" provision, the same case manager with the same physical limitation would be looked at very differently. Although he cannot perform one aspect of his job, he can perform all tasks required in the company's internal case manager position, which would not require him to leave the office. In this scenario, he may be ineligible for any benefits, or he may receive wage-loss benefits based upon the salary of the internal case manager, even if his salary as a field case manager is greater. Further, the disability insurance company's case manager may work with this employee's physician to arrange for a modified job description for the injured case manager, in which he can continue to work without traveling. This would eliminate or reduce the injured case manager's ability to receive salary replacement.

It is important to remember that disability insurance coverage is plan specific. Although the "own occ/any occ" rule exists, benefit coverage and limitations will vary depending upon the policy. Regardless of the type of coverage, the role of the disability insurance case manager is to promote early intervention, quality medical care, and customized transitional return-to-work programs, as well as to integrate disability insurance and workers' compensation benefits when available. One of the major differences between disability case management and workers' compensation case management is that the disability case manager generally cannot direct medical care, but can help control costs and outcomes by facilitating return-to-work. The disability case manager often requests that the primary care physician evaluate the functional level of the patient to explore the ability of the patient to return to gainful employment, whether at the existing job, a modified version of the job, or a different job.

WORKERS' COMPENSATION

Workers' compensation is a no-fault, individually state-governed insurance system that addresses work-related injuries and illnesses. Since 1911, when the Workers' Compensation Act was enacted (see Chapter eight), states have been mandated through employer-sponsored programs to govern wage re-placement and medical benefits for both temporary and permanent disabilities, regardless of whether the employer or the worker is at fault for the injury or illness. The goal of workers' compensation is to provide prompt medical care coordination to return the worker to gainful re-employment.

Employees are immediately covered under an employer's mandated workers' compensation insurance policy at the time of hiring. There are no waiting period or eligibility requirements. The employer is required by law to carry workers' compensation insurance for all part-time and full-time employees. Workers' compensation pays for the following if an injury or developed occupational disease occurs because of conditions related to the job:

- all reasonable and medically necessary care;
- a percentage of lost wages;
- death benefits and burial expenses to a deceased worker's dependents.

There are several differences in how medical benefits are covered under state workers' compensation programs. Some states have managed care workers' compensation systems. The managed care company directs care similar to group health managed care policies. A primary care physician evaluates the patient to determine appropriate services and whether/when the patient requires physician specialists. The managed care systems are enacted to control costs and lower variations in care. Still, many variables exist in workers' compensation systems, including how much providers can charge for certain services, and who will be an approved service provider under the reimbursement system.

The nature and extent of vocational services offered to injured workers often varies considerably based on state governance. The nature and extent of ancillary services, such as home modifications and transportation, are also very different state to state. Other variables include wage-loss compensation, such as when compensation begins, what methodology is used to determine the amount of weekly compensation, how employees report injuries to the employer, and how employers report the initial injury or event to the state system, as well as to the insurance carrier.

The intent of reporting injuries is to provide a prompt system whereby the insurance company can review the claim, investigate questionable claims, and assign a claims adjuster or claims manager to oversee the claims payment process. If case management is assigned, the case manager works closely with the claims adjuster or claims manager and is responsible to report all activity to this individual.

Nearly every state requires a waiting period for workers' compensation wage- loss benefits to begin. This circumvents compensation for minor injuries and reduces frivolous claims. A waiting period can range from three days to three weeks. If the lost time from work exceeds the waiting period, benefits are then usually paid from the date of injury. Wage-loss benefits depend upon the pre-injury earnings of the disabled worker. Each state establishes a formula so that standard benefits are determined, including a minimum and a maximum allowable benefit.

For example, in cases of total disability, the wage benefit may replace two-thirds of the worker's weekly wages. All workers' compensation wage-loss benefits are nontaxable income to the injured worker. Because workers' compensation is a return-to-work system, some states end the wage benefit at retirement age or allow a phase-out period. Wage-loss benefits under workers' compensation can be coordinated with available LTD benefits, social security disability income (SSDI), and Medicare benefits when the employee is eligible to receive these benefits. It is the responsibility of the carrier to inform the injured worker about potential benefits if the carrier suspects or confirms that the injured worker may be eligible. However, the carrier cannot reduce or withhold wage-loss benefits from the employee prior to the employee's receipt of additional benefits.

Wage-loss benefits can sometimes precipitate secondary gain. Secondary gain occurs when an employee's wage-loss benefit equals or is greater than the amount of income the employee would otherwise have when working. Because the injured worker is in a better financial situation when collecting wage-loss benefits, he/she can enjoy a *secondary gain* by not returning to work. Outside circumstances cause secondary gain. An example is the working mother with young children in day care. Although the working mother will be compensated only for two-thirds of her wages while unable to work, she is able to keep her children at home during her recovery period. The amount of money she saves is greater than the amount of money she is losing by not working. Further, she saves even more money because she does not have to drive to and from work every day. She is also able to stay home, enjoy her children, and not work. Therefore, she has a significant incentive to find ways to lengthen her necessary recovery period. In other words, she may begin to search for ways to perpetuate fraud and abuse.

Secondary gain is a challenging problem to the insurance company paying the claim, the case manager trying to return the employee to gainful employment, and the entire workers' compensation system, which suffers from an overload of fraud and abuse. Individuals with secondary gain are known as malingerers. Claims adjusters use strategies to deal with malingerers, such as hiring undercover investigative companies to observe and document activities by malingerers that would not be possible if they were as injured as they claim to be. This information is gathered in an effort to prove fraud and abuse so that the claim can be aborted.

Another difficult situation for a workers' compensation case manager is the determination of when to close a case. Some cases are ongoing for years, based on either a catastrophic injury or a chronic condition, such as a spinal cord injury, head injury, or even a low back injury. When a patient has maximized the available resources and it is believed that the patient cannot benefit from additional medical treatment, the patient is often classified as having reached "maximum medical improvement" (MMI). Only physicians trained and authorized in their respective states to determine MMI are qualified to make this determination. Oftentimes it is appropriate for a case manager to close a case when the patient has reached MMI. The claims adjuster will file a motion to close whatever aspects of the case can be legally closed once a patient has reached MMI. At this point the case manager may recommend the patient to a vocational specialist in order to continue the process of returning the patient to gainful employment, even though case management will cease. Information on rehabilitation and return-to-work is covered in Chapter 3.

There are times when a patient will reach MMI even though all medical treatment options have not been exhausted. One example of this situation would be a patient who refuses a particular surgery, even though the surgery is considered by the physician to potentially enhance the patient's physical state. The patient does not want to risk his/her health status further by consenting to the surgery. Since the surgery has been refused even though it is a viable medical treatment option, the patient can still be classified by the physician as having met MMI.

The main stakeholders in any state workers' compensation system include the employee, the employer, the insurance company, the health care providers, and the attorneys. Each has a distinctive role in this very complex system. Case managers, as part of the group of health care providers, are responsible to coordinate prompt, appropriate medical care with an end-focus of returning the individual to gainful employment. Case managers also assist the employer and the employee to prevent further injury by promoting safety in the workplace. More information on promoting safety and injury prevention in the workplace is covered in Chapter three.

Employee

Employee means any person engaged in any employment under any appointment or contract of hire or apprenticeship, express or implied, oral or written. In other words, a genuine employer-employee relationship must exist. Employees may or may not include officers of a corporation and a sole proprietor or a partner who devotes full time to the proprietorship or partnership. Employees do not include independent contractors, except that some individuals or companies may inappropriately classify and identify independent contractors in accordance with the state statutes and law for workers' compensation. In this situation the independent contractor would be covered under the workers' compensation policy of the contractor to which the independent contractor provides services. Variances in coverage of elected officers, sole proprietors, and independent contractors are due to the fact that persons in these categories may have the ability to opt out of standard coverage through a state's statutory procedures.

Employer

The employer is identified as anyone carrying on employment, and includes the legal representative of a deceased person or the receiver of trustees of any person carrying on employment. If the employer is a corporation, then all parties in actual control of the corporation, including but not limited to, the president, officers who exercise broad corporate powers, directors, and all shareholders who directly or indirectly own a controlling interest in the corporation, are considered the employer. Employer also means the state and all political subdivisions thereof, including all public and quasi-public corporations therein, including officers elected at the polls by the general voting public.

Employers almost exclusively finance state-mandated workers' compensation. By providing workers' comp coverage to their employees, employers are shielded by law from having to defend themselves against liability lawsuits filed by workers who are injured on the job. The amount of money an employer will pay for its workers' compensation policy to cover its employees is determined largely by three factors: job classifications that rate the risk of a specific job; the number of employees; and the company's accident record. Employers are primarily responsible for payments of compensation, medical services, and funeral expenses. Employers also receive guidance from state workers' compensation commissions about accident prevention and safety-in-the-workplace, which may or may not be voluntary responsibilities on the part of the employer.

Insurance Company

The insurance company acts as the payer of claims in workers' compensation. Once a state workers' compensation system has made an award of compensation to an injured worker, the payment of benefits is required by law to be made by the insurance company in a pre-determined time frame set by law. Insurance companies/carriers are responsible to make timely benefit payments to injured workers and to medical service providers of the injured worker. These include:

- medical/hospitalization benefits
- hospital and nursing services
- medicines
- crutches and other apparatus
- artificial arms, feet, hands, legs, and other prosthetic appliances
- wage reimbursement benefits

Attorneys—Plaintiff and Defense

Attorneys are legal professional representatives certified by their states to practice law. Plaintiff attorneys in the workers' compensation system represent the injured worker or the worker with an occupational illness, while defense attorneys represent the employer/carrier. In workers' compensation, the insurance company or payer is equally represented with the employer of the injured worker. Attorneys may be involved in a workers' compensation claim in matters pertaining to (but not limited to):

- whether an injury is a "covered" injury;
- whether the injured party is an employee;
- whether the injury was an accident or occupational disease;
- whether the injury arose out of employment;
- whether the injury arose in the course of the employment;
- covered benefits;
- extent of disability under the "healing" period to determine coverage.

When a case manager is involved in a workers' compensation case, interaction with the attorney is required. Before speaking to or meeting with an injured worker, the case manager must first contact the worker's attorney to gain permission to talk/meet with the worker. Many times the attorney will grant this request with no restrictions. At other times, the attorney may have restrictions and recommendations that need to be reported to the claims adjuster at the insurance company. An example of this may be that the initial meeting is held at the attorney's office. Another request from the attorney may be that the case manager copies him/her on all correspondence regarding the injured worker, including progress reports and the plan of care.

HEALTH CARE PROVIDERS

A health care provider means a physician or any recognized practitioner who provides skilled services pursuant to a prescription or under the supervision or direction of a physician, and who is recognized by the state's workers' compensation system as a health care provider. The term health care provider also includes a health care facility providing health care services. A large variety of health care providers practice within workers' compensation systems. Examples of health care professionals who are providers in a workers' compensation system may include, but not be limited to, physicians, podiatrists, chiropractors, psychologists, physician assistants, nurse practitioners, rehabilitation nurses, case managers, life-care planners, occupational therapists, physical therapists, speech therapists, rehabilitation counselors, and vocational evaluators.

AUTO LIABILITY

Like workers' compensation, auto liability insurance can provide both medical benefits and wage-loss benefits, although unlike workers' compensation, the two sets of benefits are not mandated by federal law. Like workers' compensation, there are many variables in coverage based upon the state in which the policy holder resides. Like workers' compensation, some auto liability policies are no-fault policies, covering benefits regardless of who caused the injury, although unlike workers' compensation, no-fault policies are not mandated by federal law.

In states where medical coverage is offered under auto liability policies, benefits are called personal injury protection (PIP). There are many variables of PIP, including when benefits are enacted, how long benefits are offered, and how many claims dollars can be spent. States also mandate how transition occurs when an available medical benefit is exhausted.

For example, a person injured in a motor vehicle accident by another driver may receive initial benefits for his emergency room visit under that driver's auto liability insurance coverage. However, when the at-fault driver's $5,000 major medical cap has been met, the injured driver may be responsible to assume the cost of care, or the medical benefits may be picked up by the injured person's own health insurance plan. In a no-fault auto liability system, the injured person's own auto insurance would be responsible for the payment of initial medical care until benefits are exhausted, regardless of the fact that the injured person did not cause the accident.

MANAGED CARE

Managed care as a term has come to define a broad array of systems and processes meant to control escalating health care costs while coordinating quality health care services and products through a network of approved providers. These providers, in theory, agree to assume the risk of caring for all individuals in an aggregate population for capitated, predetermined dollar amounts. Capitation is a method of payment under managed care in which the health care provider is paid a fixed amount for each person over a specific period of time, regardless of the actual number or nature of services/products provided to each person. This is known as *per member, per month*. A fixed monthly payment is provided for each member covered in the plan, regardless of whether the plan members utilize, underutilize, or overutilize the provider's services. The provider assumes the risk associated with a fixed fee.

Since 1960, and primarily since the early 1990s, employers across the U.S. have addressed increasing health care costs by replacing or supplementing their traditional indemnity health plans offered to employees with managed care plans. These plans have limited fees paid to providers and reward low rates (or penalize high rates) of service provision. Managing claims dollars spent on the aggregate is paramount to the success of a managed care organization (MCO).

In the 1970s in this country, fee-for-service, or indemnity plans were available, primarily through employer plans. Fee-for-service payments contributed to health care services that were reactively oriented—they were based upon costs stemming from injury and illness, rather than focusing on preventive measures to keep patients healthy and free from injury/illness. Costs that did have a "cap" were deeply capitated, and processes for preauthorization or concurrent review were cumbersome. In other words, predetermined fees for services and products were similar to the "reasonable and customary" costs already being charged by providers, and did not require the provider to assume any significant risk for managing the patient or authorizing the service. Thus, managed care plans were often as expensive or more expensive than fee-for-service plans, and employees were not incentivized to purchase a managed care plan.

The 1980s heralded diagnosis related groups (DRGs), requiring acute care systems to assume some risk and accountability for their lengths of stay based upon a patient's diagnosis upon admission. The concepts of managed care began to take a foothold as health care costs continued to spiral and employers struggled with increases in premiums. When the U.S. government failed to enact a universal health care system in the early 1990s, payers aggressively assumed individual responsibility to offer a menu of managed care plans to both large and small employers. To make the managed care plans affordable, payers created a paradigm shift, whereby they transposed the risk of providing quality, cost-effective care from the payer side to the provider side. This was achieved through capitation, through co-payments required of the insureds, and through limitations of coverage, including limitations or denials based upon pre-existing conditions. Since the early 1990s, federal and state governments have increasingly enacted legislation that imposes limitations on the extent of denials and control achieved by an insurance company (see Chapter eight, Managed Care Legislation section).

By the mid-1990s, it became apparent in this country that senior citizens and the poor could also benefit from a menu of managed care plans, which were being offered at various times and through various payer groups. It was determined that the elderly are particularly vulnerable to chronic conditions and require careful monitoring for effective care. Care coordination would be especially beneficial to deal with multiple practitioners, often used by these fragile groups. The elderly are excellent candidates for preventive services. Medicaid populations include high-risk pregnancies, chronicity, epidemic diseases, and limited access to care, which can greatly benefit from the care coordination offered through managed care.[1] Because managed care's focus is intended to be a wellness model, based on preventive care, fragile populations in both the Medicaid and Medicare systems could greatly benefit from this focus. Thus, a large increase in the number of managed care policies offered for Medicare and Medicaid recipients is noted in the literature during this period of time.

In 1997, the Balanced Budget Act of 1997 significantly changed how Medicare providers would be reimbursed and how Medicare consumers would receive care. The primary intent of a new program unveiled, called Medicare + Choice, was to build upon the success of the HMOs by providing additional options and encouraging further enrollment in plans separate from and different from traditional Medicare.

Despite the implementation of managed care over the past several years, debate continues as to whether managed care has provided coordination and efficiency of quality service, or has simply managed costs.[2] The management of costs has been packaged in a variety of offerings to employer groups, private pay insurance, Medicaid plans, Medicare plans, and to special group associations. Some of the most common are:

HMO

A health maintenance organization (HMO) provides health care for an aggregate in a specified geographic area. The HMO accepts responsibility for delivering an agreed-to set of services/products to an enrolled group. The HMO collects a pre-determined periodic payment paid in advance (usually on the first of each month) on behalf of each individual enrollee. Each enrollee is then responsible to assume a co-payment (usually $5–$25) that can vary in cost when seeking the services of a primary care physician, specialty physician, diagnostic center, or treatment facility. Enrollees are required to seek services from specific providers listed as the HMO's network providers. Enrollees are also required to first seek the medical attention of a pre-appointed primary care physician (classified as a gatekeeper), rather than independently assuming the need for treatment by a specialty physician. Specialty physicians, (with the usual exception of pediatricians, internists, and gynecologists) will be covered through the HMO only if the patient sees them based upon a written referral from the patient's primary care physician. They must be an authorized provider in the insurance company's network, or preauthorization for their services must have been provided by the insurance company as an out-of-network service.

The primary goal of an HMO is to enhance quality of care through a coordinated network. It is not to enhance cost savings through limitation of benefits. Yet, many accuse HMOs of rationing health care through limitation of benefits and incentivizing gatekeepers to not refer patients for treatment or specialty care. The debates will no doubt continue as HMOs continue to occupy a large share of the managed-care market.

PPO

A preferred provider organization (PPO) is a managed care system of health care delivery in which a third-party payer contracts with a group of medical care providers who furnish services at a lower-than-usual fee in return for prompt payment and a certain volume of patients. In a PPO plan, the enrollee usually has a greater list of providers to choose from in the network than in an HMO managed care plan, since providers are paid at better negotiated, capitated, or formula rates for services provided. Further, the enrollee does not need to obtain written referrals for specialty physicians from the primary care physician (gatekeeper).

In most PPO plans, an enrollee is required to pay a predetermined co-payment, or can be required to pay a percentage of the bill retrospectively (ie, payment for 10%–30% of services that have a pre-determined price tag). PPO plans cover a broad range of delivery systems. Many PPO systems are voluntary members of the American Association of Preferred Provider Organizations (AAPPO), a national nonprofit membership organization dedicated to promoting quality in PPO systems.

POS

A point-of-service plan usually offers both HMO and PPO levels of coverage, so that the enrollee has greater flexibility in choosing providers either in the managed care network, at an optimally cost-efficient fee, or outside the managed care network, in which services will still be paid, but at a reduced rate. There are many variations to POS plans offered by various insurers. Many are open-access HMOs, whereby the guidelines of an HMO apply, but without a confined network of providers from which to choose. Some have the guidelines of a PPO, but limit access to specialty physicians by requiring a referral from the primary (gatekeeper) physician. Another version may allow open access into and out of a network, but will impose financial penalties for stepping outside the network.

IPA

An Independent Practice Association (IPA) is an HMO that contracts in a risk-sharing or full-risk arrangement with physicians. The physicians still see patients in their own private offices, and are reimbursed on a capitated basis.

Looking at managed care from a tongue-in-cheek point of view, remember when:

- Doctors were doctors and not providers?
- Patients weren't members or subscribers?
- A network was one of three television companies offering you a choice of programs?
- Covered lives were customers?
- A gatekeeper was someone hired to secure property?

THIRD PARTY ADMINISTRATOR

A third-party administrator (TPA) engages in claims administration service contracts with self-funded companies and employer groups. TPAs assume administrative responsibility at a fixed rate to handle all claims; to process claims; to handle all customer correspondence, complaints, appeals, etc; and to act as a liaison between the payer and the provider groups. TPAs are able to undertake the heavy paperwork, care coordination and documentation systems that self-funded groups are often not equipped or financially able to handle. Many insureds employ TPAs to act as their claims administration arm. Case managers often report to TPAs because the TPA is responsible to manage those aspects of care coordination that the case manager influences—cost, quality, and access to care.

MEDICARE

Medicare is a federally funded government program that was enacted by federal legislation in 1965, and is administered by the Centers for Medicare and Medicaid Services (CMS) within the US Department of Health and Human Services (HHS). Most people age 65 and older are entitled to free Medicare Part A, which is considered hospital insurance. Part A covers inpatient hospital services, skilled nursing facilities, approved home health services, and hospice care. Persons eligible for Medicare include those eligible for Social Security Income (SSI) retirement benefits, those eligible for Railroad Retirement benefits, and those under 65 who have been eligible for Social Security Disability Income (SSDI) benefits for at least 24 months. Examples include the person with a mental impairment, a catastrophic illness, or a chronic illness. Persons may claim Medicare 24 months after the date of injury or after the illness is diagnosed and documented by a physician. There is a 5-month waiting period for persons seeking eligibility. A "fast track" application process exists for persons diagnosed with a terminal illness who are considered to have 6 months or less to live. Persons under age 65 who have kidney disease that "appears irreversible and permanent and requires a regular course of dialysis or kidney transplantation to maintain life" are also eligible for free Part A Medicare.

Medicare Part A recipients are automatically eligible for Medicare Part B (medical insurance), providing they can pay the designated monthly premiums established through insurance companies providing Part B insurance. Part B covers physician services, outpatient hospital services, medical equipment and supplies. Premiums for Part B insurance vary widely, particularly because some Part B policies are fee-for-service, or indemnity plans, and some are managed care plans. Senior citizens may have excellent Part B coverage, more limited managed care coverage, or no Part B coverage at all. Through a managed care plan they may have some coverage for prescriptions, under a "prescription card coverage", in which they may be responsible for a co-pay on prescription drugs. Under the Medicare Prescription Drug, Improvement and Modernization Act (MMA) of 2003, seniors and people living with disabilities were provided with a voluntary prescription drug benefit through Medicare effective in 2006. The intent of the MMA is to offer more choices and better benefits. In fact, approval of the MMA represented the most significant improvement to senior health care in nearly 40 years. Passage of the MMA was also intended to offer more health plan choices, including regional preferred provider organizations (PPOs), to provide better benefits, higher quality care, and substantial cost savings for Medicare beneficiaries.

In addition to the standard drug benefit, which is available to all beneficiaries with a 75 percent premium subsidy, passage of the MMA provided low-income seniors and people with a disability who have limited means—about a third of all people with Medicare—with greater access to coverage offering limited premiums and deductibles and no gaps in coverage. Medicare beneficiaries with retiree coverage benefited from a set of options to obtain more affordable enhanced coverage, including a new retiree drug subsidy as well as options for employers and unions to wrap around Medicare coverage or offer Medicare-subsidized drug coverage themselves. In addition, states, other individuals, and charitable organizations can contribute towards a beneficiary's out-of-pocket costs and still have those contributions count towards catastrophic coverage.

Initially under Medicare, physicians under Part B were paid at a "usual and customary fee" for a particular service. When DRGs were unveiled in late 1993, physicians began receiving payments under a Resource Based Relative Value Scale (RBRVS) system. Hospitals began being paid through the Prospective Payment System (PPS), which used the DRG process and formulas. DRG payments were based largely upon diagnosis and expected length of stay, so that physicians were no longer incentivized to keep their patients in the hospital. As hospital systems became more astute at collaborating with their physicians for aggressive discharge planning, costs were reduced significantly. Managed care plans in the 1990s have assumed the risk of Medicare to target similar cost savings through their managed care Part B plans. Some plans are successful, while others announce "an end" to covering Medicare lives based on significant losses in managing this often fragile population.

MEDICAID

Another fragile population is the Medicaid population, which is served through joint federal and state programs and varies in covered benefits state-to-state. Medicaid was enacted in 1965 under Title XIX of the Social Security Act. Eligibility for Medicaid is based on income and other financial resources of the applicant. In addition to financial need, an individual may qualify for Medicaid based on medical need, as well as categorical need, meaning that the person is already receiving some form of government benefits, such as Social Security Income (SSI). If a child is under the age of 21 and has an impairment severe enough to meet the disability standards under SSI, the parental income is disregarded in determining Medicaid benefits.

The provision of Medicaid benefits can vary somewhat from state to state, although in all states Medicaid will pay for skilled home health care nursing services, as well as for long-term care in a nursing home, provided financial minimal requirements are met. Within broad guidelines established by the federal government, each state sets criteria for its Medicaid program, including:

- Eligibility standards
- Type, amount, duration, and scope of eligible services
- Rate of payment for services offered
- Administration of the program

MUTUAL AND INDEMNITY

Mutual and indemnity plans refer to traditional profit-making, premium-based insurance companies where reimbursement or compensation for loss or personal injury is provided via a contract that is preset and includes premiums. Companies selectively purchase these policies in much the same way as individuals would purchase homeowners' or automobile insurance. Indemnity group and individual health insurance plans were quite common in the 1960s, 1970s and even the 1980s, until their annual increases in premiums became more than insureds could manage, and masses of people turned to managed care plans offering lower premiums.

Indemnity plans largely reimburse for services based on a "usual and customary charge", and then use these pre-set charges to calculate payment of a majority percentage of the total bill, usually about 80%. Payments are made retrospectively, so that if a provider is not willing to "accept assignment"—that is, to accept direct payment from the indemnity plan without collecting funds from the insured at the time services are rendered—the insured will then be responsible to pay the bill in full, and seek a portion of reimbursement from the insurance company. Providers can also require the insured to pay the stated percentage he/she is personally responsible to cover under the plan (20% or 30% are customary percentages) up front, or in installments. The provider then bills the insurance company, obtaining payment for services under a "reasonable and customary" formula, which may or may not be equal to the amount billed.

INTEGRATED DELIVERY SYSTEMS

Integrated delivery systems (IDS) emerged in the 1990s as a method of "risk sharing" under contract with managed care organizations. In an IDS system, services provided range from the acute to the post-acute continuum of care, and all are integrated. This system was established primarily to:

- share the risk of capitation, spreading the risk across several entities to hedge against a loss in any one delivery system;
- maximize available funding and benefits coverage from the pay source;
- move the patient through the continuum of care in a seamless system;
- enhance coordinated care delivery by ensuring that the patient's care is communicated and coordinated between various delivery systems.

Patients in an IDS system were formerly moved through the integrated system by discharge planners, without regard for offering the patient choices in other available post-acute services outside the IDS. The federal government circumvented this practice in the latter part of the 1990s when it prevented entities accepting Medicare from self-referring patients to integrated post-acute services within the IDS, without offering the patient choices of other service providers.

IDS systems continue to evolve to meet the needs of patients who are being discharged quicker and sicker from acute care settings. Case managers are also developing more sophisticated resource management models in IDS systems, particularly as an effective strategy to avoid the pitfalls of self-referral. More information on resource management is covered under Chapter five.

MILITARY HEALTH SYSTEM

The U.S. Military Health Service System (MHSS), formerly known as Champus, uses a managed care delivery system known as TRICARE. TRICARE was initiated to manage the rising costs of health care in the military system. TRICARE is operated under the Department of Defense and is the nation's largest health care system with more than 8.3 million individuals eligible to receive care. All active duty military personnel, their families, retirees and their families, and survivors of active duty military personnel who are not eligible for Medicare based upon age can participate in one of three levels of TRICARE. Additionally, individuals under the age of 65 who are eligible for Medicare because of disability and end-stage renal disease may also choose to participate.

The three levels of TRICARE are TRICARE Prime, TRICARE Standard, and TRICARE Extra. All active duty men and women are automatically enrolled in TRICARE Prime. The focus of TRICARE Prime is to keep the enrollees "fit for duty". In this regard, TRICARE Prime leads the nation in providing a coordinated, system-wide wellness program. TRICARE Prime uses a strong case management and disease management approach to support its wellness and illness/injury prevention model. Other military eligible individuals can choose among the Prime, Standard, and Extra levels of TRICARE. Once retired military personnel, their families, and survivors reach 65, they are eligible under Medicare and are not usually eligible for TRICARE.[3]

VOCATIONAL REHABILITATION

Vocational Rehabilitation (VR) is provided state-to-state, with eligibility criteria set by individual states in accordance with federal law. In general, to be eligible for services provided through state VR programs, persons must have a physical or mental impairment that impedes employment; and must be reasonably expected to become employable as a result of services provided. In this regard, a disabled child who is not nearing the employment age of 16 would not be eligible for VR services. Likewise, a disabled individual over the retirement age of 70 would not be eligible. The intent is to address the individual's physical, mental, behavioral and environmental needs so that successful, gainful employment can be achieved, moving the disabled person to self-reliance and independence.

VR is often termed "the payer of last resort". In addition to funding medical services, it provides training and education for individuals who otherwise have little or no medical and/or vocational coverage. Services provided include:

- vocational training
- secondary education necessary to achieve appropriate employment. (These might include an associate degree from a school of nursing or a bachelor's degree in computer technology.)
- financial support during rehabilitation
- communication services (ie, readers and note-takers to assist a blind candidate while in a school or training institution funded by VR)
- physical and mental rehabilitation services (ie, acute and post-acute medical care; prosthetic and assistive devices; transportation; home and jobsite modifications for independence; therapies, such as OT, PT, speech.

LONG-TERM CARE

Although long-term care is covered in Chapter one as a health care setting, it is also a reimbursement system that is gaining momentum in our aging environment. Long-term care (LTC) insurance provides one of the only options for supportive care available to the older population. Medicare provides limited LTC benefits for up to 120 days per year. Patients requiring extended care coverage beyond this timeframe are faced with the difficulty of paying costs out of their own pockets. Medicare's coverage is intended to assist the patient who requires an extended recovery period following an illness or injury, but does not need the intensive care of a hospital for the recovery. It is not intended to provide ongoing residential nursing home care.

Most private health insurance plans do not include LTC coverage as a standard provision. Medicaid is a large provider of LTC, but only for the poor who are eligible for coverage. For the younger population, LTC insurance can be vitally important if a catastrophic injury occurs. The spinal cord injured patient's health insurance policy limits rehabilitation coverage and provides very limited or no custodial care benefit. Yet, the spinal cord injured patient may require lifelong assistance.

Formerly, LTC insurance provided only nursing home care, but today's expanded health care arena allows many services potentially covered under LTC insurance. These may include:

- hospice
- adult day care centers
- sub-acute or skilled nursing facilities
- transitional living centers
- home health care and custodial care

Case managers working with patients possessing LTC insurance policies must be aware of the level of service provided in the policy—skilled care, intermediate, or custodial. If the plan does cover custodial care, the patient may be covered only if cognitive deficits are present, or two or more activities of daily living (ADLs) are impaired. These are called "benefit triggers", which define the clinical conditions that must be present in order for the insured to receive benefits. A policy will state how many ADLs (usually at least two) must be deficient and to what degree before the policy benefits take effect. Cognitive impairments are defined as a deficiency in either short-term or long-term memory as to person, place or time, or deducive or abstract reasoning.

Some contracts also allow for medical necessity, which permits an insured to access benefits if s/he does not meet the ADL or cognitive impairment standard.[4] Under medical necessity, a physician or other health care professional can certify that the requested care is correct and appropriate to the insured's care. Often, LTC plans use their own case managers or contracted case managers to make this determination. The case manager will visit the policy holder in his/her home, assessing the patient's health status, and functional and cognitive needs. Needs for ADL assistance are noted. The determination for benefits will be based largely upon this comprehensive assessment.

REFERENCES

1. Moreo, K. Newest case management strategies of managed care organizations. *Journal of Care Management.* 1999: 5,6:10–19.
2. Feder & Moon. Managed care for the elderly: a threat or a promise? *Generations: Journal of the American Society on Aging.* 1998: 6,7:23–24.
3. TRICARE. Department of Defense Health Affairs Department. Washington, D.C.: U.S. Government Printing Office. 1996.
4. Moreo, K. *Disability management and rehabilitation specialist handbook.* Miramar, FL: Professional Resources In Management Education, Inc. 2000: 87–90.

LEGAL AND ETHICAL ISSUES 10

Case managers working in every health care setting have increasing responsibility to make cost-effective decisions that are ethical and legally defensible.[1] To understand how to make ethical and legally defensible decisions, case managers must understand the difference between ethics and legal compliance. Legal compliance is based upon rules of conduct established and enforced by authority to prohibit extremes in behavior. These rules have strategies to prevent, detect and punish legal violations of the rules. Legal compliance is unlikely to include moral commitment or to inspire human excellence.[2] Ethics is a science that deals with principles of right or wrong; good or bad. Ethics governs our relationships with others. It is a value-based, integrity-based strategy of adherence to moral principles and character. It is based on personal beliefs and values which guide our decision-making process. Ethics are broader, deeper and more demanding than legal compliance because they require an active effort to define responsibility and action.

From an ethical standpoint, case managers are challenged to consistently do the right thing for the patient while balancing cost constraints and limited resources. As proclaimed patient advocates, case managers focus on advancing the welfare of patients, but these patients are served by a complex array of health care delivery systems with varying degrees of economic constraints. Further, the role of advocacy can often be in direct conflict with legal responsibility, particularly when case managers are making initial determinations regarding authorization for services or payment.[3]

Advocacy is a fundamental ethical responsibility of case management. It is demanded in guidelines for professional conduct upheld by national case management certifications. It is governed by case managers' professional licensing boards, such as individual states' nurse practice acts. It is written into case management job descriptions. It appears in standards of practice authored by national membership organizations. For example, the *Code of Ethics* and the *Standards of Clinical Nursing Practice* by the American Nurses Association (ANA) cite the nurse as a client advocate. These are applied in nursing case management. The CMSA *Standards of Practice for Case Management* cites advocacy as a key role of the case manager, regardless of discipline:

> The client's best interests are represented by the case manager's advocacy for necessary funding, treatment alternatives, timelines and coordination of health services, and frequent re-evaluation of progress and goals.[4]

To balance advocacy with the limitations of payers and resources, case managers need to draw on the skills discussed in the opening chapter. Empowering the patient and family to become involved in decisions regarding treatments and services promotes advocacy. Communicating effectively with all members of the health care team, including the patient and family, promotes relationship-building. Being truthful and fair when working with the patient/family and the payer promotes appropriate decision-making. These skills are part of the moral principles governing ethics, known as ethical principles.

ETHICAL PRINCIPLES

Ethical principles serve as guidelines for case managers in daily practice. These include the five moral principles of autonomy, beneficence, nonmaleficence, justice, and veracity. Each case manager is responsible to understand the obligations and duties as a case manager, and to incorporate moral principles into daily practice. To accomplish this, case managers in every job setting should begin by objectively judging their ability to practice ethically in their employment.[5] One way to accomplish this is to consider the following questions:

- What is expected of me as an employee?
- Is my job description in conflict with my own moral beliefs?
- Am I expected to make compromises in the best interest of my employer, and if so, are there alternatives if these decisions compromise my ethical practice?
- Is cost containment the bottom line, and if so, to what extent am I expected to control costs?
- Are there processes in place to make exceptions for patients who need services/products that may cost more money?
- Are there processes in place for objective decisions to be made regarding patient care?
- Is quality measured by the employer, and are there written policies and procedures in place for continuous quality improvement?
- Will I be provided with opportunities for continuing education to advance my professional knowledge in the field?

If the case manager determines that the ability exists to practice ethically in the employment setting, moral principles must then be applied to the case manager's daily practice.

Autonomy

Autonomy is the moral principle governing a person's right to make his or her own decisions. It is respect for others and for their uniqueness. In health care, the patient should be encouraged to make decisions about his/her health care treatment, even if the decisions are difficult for health care providers to accept. The principle of autonomy is evident in the Patient Self-Determination Act of 1990 (see Chapter eight), a law prompted by the needs of patients to determine in advance whether they desire life-supporting measures should they become incapacitated by injury or illness. Autonomy promotes independence and gives the patient an inherent right to determine what happens according to his/her own preferences and value system.

Beneficence

Beneficence is the moral principle governing a person's obligation to promote good, to further a person's legitimate interests, and to actively prevent or remove harm. Beneficence requires the case manager to promote the well-being of the patient/family within the constraints of the health care system. This includes using good resource management skills to promote a safe discharge for a patient. If an elderly female patient with a fractured hip has no one at home to assist her with ADLs, that patient can be at risk of falling. A wheelchair-bound patient cannot safely be discharged to a home environment that has steps and narrow doorways. Information on how to promote safe discharges through resource management is covered in Chapter five.

Nonmaleficence

Nonmaleficence means to refrain from doing harm to others. Case managers can gauge nonmaleficence by understanding and incorporating outcome measurements into their daily practice. Outcomes can provide a picture about the quality, cost, and appropriateness of care delivered to a patient. Information on outcome measurements is covered in Chapter four. More formal methods of governing nonmaleficence are provided through ethics committees established in many health care settings. Ethics committees are intended to provide an objective means to promote nonmaleficence and other forms of ethical practice. Ethics committees are particularly active in acute care settings, where ethical dilemmas often arise surrounding such issues as high-tech medical care, advance directives, conflicting wishes of family members, mental competence of patients, surrogacy, and unsafe discharges or transfers. The roles of ethics committees include educating, informing, advising and deciding.

Justice

Justice is defined as maintaining what is right and fair. It is the moral principle that governs the responsibility of the case manager to coordinate appropriate allocation of resources to meet the patient's health care needs. It is a moral principle that, when practiced consistently, can establish and promote trust between the patient and the case manager. Case managers should also practice justice when collaborating with other members of the health care team, including working with payers and providers. If a case manager considers what is right and fair before making decisions and recommendations about health care services and resources, he/she is practicing the golden rule—doing unto others as you would have them do unto you. This will clearly promote trust by others in the actions and in the intent of the case manager.

Veracity

Veracity is truth-telling, and it also is an important component of developing a trusting relationship with the patient, family, providers, and payers. In today's health care climate, there exists an unfortunate element of mistrust among many patients who are confused by a convoluted health care delivery system. Further, physicians often mistrust payers. Health care professionals often mistrust each other's actions. Overall, it is sometimes a difficult climate in which to promote trust-building for the patient who is most vulnerable during illness or injury. Veracity can promote trust and enhance trusting relationships.

Advocacy vs. Paternalism

This chapter and others have discussed advocacy in case management; yet, there are times and situations in health care delivery when case managers can easily confuse advocacy with paternalism, resulting in an ethical dilemma. Paternalism occurs when an outside person assumes a "parental role" in making decisions that are perceived to be in the best interest of another person, without consulting the person for approval.

An example of paternalism is when the case manager develops a care plan for a patient without involving the patient or family in the care plan, believing he/she knows what is in the best interest of the patient. The case manager might arrange for an AIDS patient to participate in a community support group as part of a discharge plan, yet the patient has no intention of talking to strangers about her illness and is angry that the case manager did not consult her first. Although the case manager in advocating for the patient's best interests, failing to involve the patient in decisions about care erases advocacy and promotes paternalism. Paternalism promotes mistrust, miscommunication, and a general breakdown in the relationship. It is an easy mistake to make, and one that case managers can innocently commit if they fail to place the patient/family at the center of care decisions.

CLIENT/PATIENT RIGHTS

Patients have many rights promoted by ethical practice and promulgated by legislation. Several laws and acts have been enacted in the U.S. to protect the rights of patients and persons in the health care system, and many of them are covered in Chapter eight. Patient rights are protected under such well-known health care legislative acts as the Health Insurance Portability and Accountability Act (HIPAA), which most recently released mandates to protect patient confidentiality; the Patient Self-Determination Act, promoting a patient's right to accept or refuse treatment should they become gravely ill or injured; and the Emergency Medical Treatment and Active Labor Act (EMTLA), protecting patients from being refused emergency medical treatment.

Patient rights in health care are also promoted through ethical practice, as explored earlier in this chapter. The Patient Bill of Rights was created under President Clinton's administration to address the rights of patients in managed care. Patient rights are addressed by state boards of medicine, nursing, social work, and many other health care professional boards. Patient rights are publicly posted by hospitals in compliance with the Joint Commission on the Accreditation of Hospitals (JCAHO). In short, consideration of "the right" of individuals to have health care rights has been explored for years in nearly every facet of health care delivery. This is because society has a fundamental belief that every person has a right to basic health care. As was discussed in Chapter two, health care has been considered a fundamental right for generations. It has been argued that the right to access health care is addressed in the original Bill of Rights because, without the ability to attain or sustain wellness, the rights to life, liberty, and the pursuit of happiness become meaningless in the wake of ignorance, pain, illness and disease.[6]

Since that time, the fundamental right to access health care has been proclaimed by accreditation bodies, organizations, global alliances, presidential committees, and even the Constitution of the World Health Organization. In 1972, the American Nurses' Association officially endorsed the 1948 United Nations Universal Declaration of Human Rights, which includes the right to access health care.

PROVIDER'S RIGHTS

The focus of rights in health care is largely spent on patients and consumers. However, providers of health care also are protected by many of the same ethical and legal provisions that protect patients. For example, each of the ethical principles discussed in this chapter also applies to moral behavior toward providers. Consider the ethical principle of justice. Case managers are ethically bound to treat the providers with whom they are negotiating in a just manner—doing what is right and fair. This means that the case manager doesn't disclose one provider's bid for services/products to a competing provider in order to ensure that the second provider presents a lower bid. This action may benefit the payer and may make the case manager's cost-savings outcome appear favorable, but it is unethical behavior. In this regard, practicing ethically protects the provider's rights to a fair bid process. Case managers should apply the ethical principle of veracity when communicating, collaborating and negotiating with providers of health care services and products. This builds relationships, strengthens the likelihood of a positive outcome for the patient, and protects the provider's right to have objective, factual information.

From a legal standpoint, there are times when providers' rights are protected because it is apparent that the provider is acting in a good-faith effort on behalf of the patient. For example, most states uphold the right of a hospital and its health care personnel to treat a minor patient without a parent's written consent, when the child is suspected of being the victim of child abuse. In this case, both the hospital and its personnel are considered providers of health care and will likely be protected from legal liability because treatment is necessary and consent not possible.

Another example is the due process of proving malpractice which initially protects the provider from frivolous claims. Patients claiming malpractice of a provider in a court of law must prove negligence. The proof of negligence has four points that place the onus of proof on the patient, or claimant, to demonstrate that the provider was negligent in actions. This will be explained later in the chapter under the section on "malpractice". A final example can be demonstrated by considering the Emergency Medical Treatment and Active Labor Act (EMTLA), which protects the rights of all patients to receive a medical screening and to receive emergency treatment. This law also protects providers by ensuring that, when the acute care facility provides the medical screening, it is reimbursed for the service by the insurance company.

DELEGATION OF CARE

The EMTALA, known as the "patient dumping law", also addresses delegation of care, as explained in Chapter eight. Specific law mandates that when a patient is eligible for transfer to another facility for necessary care, legal guidelines determine delegation of care from one facility to another. Internally, health care facilities and systems must determine how delegation of care will occur in an ethical and legal manner, and then set policies and procedures to govern appropriate delegation of care. Entire patient management processes are developed and job descriptions molded to ensure that the delegation of care is purposeful and appropriate.

Delegation is a contractual agreement in which authority and responsibility for a task is transferred by the person accountable for the task to another individual. When performed appropriately, delegation benefits the delegator, the delegatee, the organization, and the patient. Appropriate delegation involves all of the following components:

- identifying and determining the task and the level of responsibility;
- identifying who has the skills and abilities to delegate;
- describing expectations clearly;
- reaching a mutual agreement on the assigned task or duties;
- equipping the delegatee with the resources to carry out the assigned task or duties;
- monitoring the performance of the delegatee and providing feedback when necessary.

Adhering to the steps of delegation minimizes the risk of liability to a health care professional, particularly if the health care professional prudently selects a qualified person as the delegatee, and provides appropriate supervision of performance. This is notably true in case management, where delegation of care can also pertain to appropriate assignment of services and products to benefit a patient.

If an infant is born with severe congenital abnormalities, care for the infant in the first year could be so intense that claims use up nearly all available coverage, leaving no funding for the child at age 3, or 6, or 12, or 18. The pediatric case manager's responsibility will be to manage the infant's benefits, tapping into community resources and eligible social services early, to preserve benefits for as long as possible. Delegation in this regard implies an ability to identify and use services and products that ensure quality, cost-effective care for the infant.

Case managers sometimes aren't as organized about delegating care once responsibility for the patient reaches their department. Case managers often fail to delegate care once they have initiated a care plan and are coordinating services. Instead of consulting with a dietician and a social worker for the non-compliant adolescent diabetic, the case manager tries to sort through the teenager's anger over being "sick" and refusal to eat the right foods.

Why does the case manager fail to follow through with delegation? Good case management requires the professional to be very proficient. Many case managers have a "just do it" attitude. They try to be all things to all people. Others see delegation as a loss of control. Still others are mistrustful that the task will be completed in a timely and efficient manner by someone else. It is important for the case manager to differentiate which tasks should be completed by a case manager, and which should be completed by other professionals, by the caregiver or even by the patient. The best interests of the patient should be the deciding factor when considering delegation.[7]

DOCUMENTATION

Documentation is the thread that connects all of the complex processes of patient care coordination in all health care settings. Every health care professional is responsible to document involvement in a patient's care; response to care; mutually planned goals for optimal recovery/wellness; issues/concerns that arise during care delivery or coordination to meet those goals; and evaluation of goals and outcomes. These responsibilities are personified when the health care professional is the case manager, since the case manager is responsible for overall care coordination. If the case manager's involvement in a patient's care includes required compliance with state or federal laws, the case manager should also document that the work was conducted within the guidelines of the federal or state law(s).

Documentation by the case manager is critical to provide a fluid picture of the patient's journey through the continuum of care. Documented information should be objective. It should present an accurate picture of health status, as well as the prognosis and goals. Documentation should be free of suspicion, conjectures, and allegations, since documents are legally discoverable and can be subpoenaed.

When working with providers, the case manager should require all providers to submit documentation on a periodic basis. The documentation should be clear and concise, and should detail the provider's plan of care, the patient's response to the plan of care, the patient's understanding of the plan of care, and the goals that are being met. Pertinent information should be shared with the treating physician to assist him/her in determining further treatment, as well as recognizing the ability of the patient to assume normal or modified activities, such as a return to work.

Payer-based case managers document their activities and incorporate providers' documentation within the patient care plan. The care plan is available to identified authorities within the payer organization, as well as to the treating physician and other members of the health care team when appropriate. The care plan must also be available to the patient upon request (see the section on Confidentiality later in this chapter) or the patient's attorney, if any. Provider-based case managers submit their documentation to identified authorities within the provider organization along with the payer case manager, the treating physician when appropriate, other members of the health care team when appropriate, and the patient or the patient's attorney.

ADVANCE DIRECTIVES

Advance directives are generally known as living wills and are governed by laws in most states under a variety of names. They are legal documents directed by a competent individual, intended to allow the individual to determine and control the degree of medical treatment and life-sustaining measures to be initiated when the individual's death is imminent. An example of a patient's intent to direct and control the degree of medical treatment administered is a "do not resuscitate" order, also know as a DNR. Case managers are responsible to be familiar with the scope of the law on advance directives in states where they practice, since health care professionals are responsible to implement advance directives on the patient's behalf. Advance directives are intended to remove all questions and doubt from family members and health care practitioners regarding the treatment wishes of the individual.

Most advance directives allow an individual to designate another individual to serve as his/her health care representative or health care surrogate in the event the individual becomes incompetent. Advance directives in most states can be revoked at any time orally or in writing, and usually become legal when provided to the individual's physician or a health care facility. The legal age for a person to complete an advance directive varies from state to state, with the minimal age generally being 18.

Because there is variation in state laws regarding the creation, enforcement, and interpretation of advance directives, case managers must understand the law in their individual state. Facility-based case managers should know the facility's policies and procedures for securing an advance directive, and the role of the case manager. Case managers should also be vigilant in reviewing the charts of patients assigned to case management to ensure that the presence of an advance directive is documented. Any discussion with the patient regarding the advance directive in place should be documented. If the patient tells the case manager that he/she wishes to rescind the advance directive, the case manager must follow the facility's policies and procedures in reporting this information to the proper authorities.[8]

AGGRESSIVE vs. PALLIATIVE CARE

There is often a fine line that differentiates when a physician will initiate aggressive medical care and when a physician will determine that palliative care is most appropriate for a patient. An investigation published in the *Annals of Internal Medicine* in 1996 found that physicians generally were more likely to issue DNR orders for patients over the age of 75. The study concluded that age was not a factor in the physicians' decisions. Rather, the study concluded that physicians are doing a better job of honoring the wishes of their elderly patients than in prior years, although they may treat younger patients overaggressively. The authors of the study theorized that it may be easier for physicians to speak to elderly patients more frankly about the possibility of dying, rather than to younger patients, whom they are less willing to let die.[9] In studying more than 10,000 patients from five medical centers over a nine-year period, the researchers determined that great variability existed in the use of DNR orders. Intensive care physicians were most likely to use DNRs (36%), while cardiologists were least likely to issue DNR orders (22%).

Case managers are also faced with the issue of aggressive versus palliative care in dealing with patients. A classic example is the cancer patient. The case manager may not have a problem talking to the elderly cancer patient about his choice of palliative care over surgery and chemotherapy. If the patient's leg tumor requires amputation and aggressive adjuvant therapy, it is easy to understand how palliative care could be a better quality of life choice. But would the case manager feel the same way about the patient's choice of palliative care if the patient were a young professional tennis player? Conversely, it may seem appropriate to amputate the young professional tennis player's leg to save a life but would this choice be made for an 80-year-old cancer victim?

When a case manager is first outlining the goals of treatment for a patient, there is an ethical duty to speak with the patient, or ensure that another member of the health care team has spoken with the patient to discuss the goals of therapy. In the case of a cancer patient, the goals of therapy may be to:

- Cure: Arrest the cancer by eradicating the malignancy.
- Control: Prolong survival and optimize functional capacity by administering therapies that will induce remission for as long as possible.
- Palliative care: Reduce/stop the patient's suffering and maximize the quality of life.

Central to palliative or end-of-life care is the use of pain management with opiate drugs such as morphine, analgesics, and a calculated pain control regimen; and, the use of hospice to offer medical and psychological support. Quality of life goals in palliative care include relief of symptoms, control of side effects, comfort measures, a focus on easing anxiety and fear, and assistance to prepare the patient and family for acceptance of death. Case managers cannot be effective in coordinating palliative care or assisting the patient/family through the end-of-life phase unless they are comfortable with their own concepts of death and dying. Case managers need to incorporate death care into their professional practice by making a commitment to obtain knowledge regarding resources, services, and products available to assist the patient and family during the final phase of life.

LEGAL RESPONSIBILITIES

In addition to the many ethical issues and ethical dilemmas facing case managers in professional practice, there are many legal responsibilities that are a common part of case management practice. The first of these to be discussed is legal responsibility surrounding patient abandonment.

Abandonment

Unfortunately, abandonment of patients occurs in many settings and for a myriad of reasons. Case managers may be exposed to newborns who have been abandoned by their parent(s) and require immediate medical care in addition to urgent application for social services, such as parental foster care and ongoing medical coverage. The case manager or resource manager will initially concentrate on mobilizing services to provide the infant with the most basic needs—food, shelter, and safety—while at the same time following the organization's legal procedures pertaining to abandonment, which is in compliance with individual state laws on abandonment. These may include cooperating with local authorities in an attempt to identify one or both parents in order to collect medical or other background information that could be vital to the infant's future well-being.

Similarly, many challenges surround abandoned adults, particularly developmentally disabled adults and older individuals. Adults can be abandoned in their own homes or in adult-care homes and facilities since abandonment does not necessarily mean that a caregiver has permanently left the premises.

Abandonment is the willful neglect of responsibility for another person by an individual who is assigned to care for that person or by an individual who is in a caregiving position. When an infant is abandoned at a police station by the parent, the intent of abandonment is clear. Abandonment of an older, ill, or injured individual being cared for by a third party is more difficult to define. Abandonment should be suspected if:

- the caregiver leaves for a period of time without arranging for substitute care;
- an employed aide does not show up for work;
- an individual's care deteriorates markedly, even with the presence of the caregiver in the home or facility.[10]

There are times when case managers may observe older patients or developmentally disabled patients who are transferred to a hospital from a caregiver setting and appear neglected or abused. The patient may have serious bedsores, wounds, bruises, emaciation, or other signs of physical neglect or abuse. Acute care facilities have policies and procedures in place to report any suspicion of abuse or neglect. The case manager should be familiar with these policies and procedures to uphold the right of the patient, as well as the legal responsibility of the case manager and the facility.

Whether abandonment is legal or illegal, and what punishment, if any, will be applied, depends on individual state law. Again, it is the responsibility of the case manager to know and understand the law(s) of the state in which the case manager practices since each state is unique in its legislation. A number of states in the U.S. have passed laws permitting parents to drop off babies at specified "safe places", such as hospitals and police stations, with no questions asked and no penalties enforced. These laws are intended to protect mothers who might otherwise harm or abandon their unwanted babies. Laws pertaining to abandonment of older persons also vary state to state, and are usually captured under the umbrella of elder abuse.

Reporting of Abuse

Elder abuse and child abuse are unfortunate and often occur in devastating circumstances to which the case manager will likely be exposed from time to time. In addition to the many services the case manager may mobilize on behalf of an abused patient, case managers and all health care professionals are legally responsible to report any suspicion of abuse. Again, each state varies in the laws pertaining to abuse and the reporting of abuse. Case managers must be familiar with the state laws governing the reporting of abuse for their practice or in which the patient resides. They must also be familiar with policies and procedures of their employers regarding the reporting of abuse within a health care facility.

Reporting of both child and elder abuse is mandatory in many states for *any person* who suspects or has reason to suspect abuse. However, every state and the District of Columbia have statutes identifying mandatory reporters of child maltreatment, and under what circumstances they are to report.[11] Individuals typically identified as mandatory reporters include all health care practitioners, law enforcement or social service agency employees, any dependent care custodian or provider, coroners, and school personnel. Failure to report abuse is punishable.

How and where to report suspected abuse varies according to state law. If a case manager suspects abuse, he/she should know the hotline 800 numbers to report abuse within all 50 states. This information is readily available in health care facilities, such as in emergency rooms of acute care hospitals. Hotline numbers are also available in various web sites on the Internet. Elder abuse hot lines for all 50 states are listed under http://alzheimers. about.com, and for children under the National Clearinghouse on Child Abuse and Neglect Information at http://nccanch.acf.gov. Generally, the same laws that require persons to report abuse protect individuals from criminal liability for reporting the suspected abuse, unless the individual reporting the abuse knowingly makes false statements. The identity of the person reporting the abuse is kept confidential.

Informed Consent

The basis of informed consent is the belief that a patient has a right to determine what will be done with his or her own body. Legally, it is a well established principle that all health care professionals are responsible to make adequate disclosures of information to a patient and to obtain an informed consent from the patient. The person who is legally responsible to obtain informed consent is the person who will provide the treatment or service to the patient. In case management, this means that a written consent must be obtained from the patient before case management services can be provided. The process to obtain an informed consent may be provided by the facility or organization where the case manager is employed, or may be obtained directly by the case manager. It is the case manager's responsibility to know and follow the process for obtaining informed consent at his/her place of employment.

To carry out the legal steps involved in informed consent, the following requirements must be met when obtaining informed consent from a patient or family member:

- Capacity: Ensure that the person consenting is competent and of legal age to consent;
- Voluntariness: Ensure that the person consenting is exercising freedom of choice without force, fraud, deceit, duress, or coercion;
- Information: Ensure that the information provided is understandable by the person consenting.

Information provided should include:

- Explanation of treatment;
- Expected results, including chances of success or failure;
- Possible risks and discomforts;
- Possible benefits;
- Possible alternatives to achieve the desired results;
- Likely medical consequences without any treatment at all.

In addition to the above steps, informed consent means that the health care professional answers any questions the patient may have and allows the patient to withdraw consent at any time. The informed consent should be witnessed by a second objective individual who can attest to the fact that the patient is informed.

Informed consent can be actual or implied. Actual consent means that the health care professional has explained the risks, the alternative procedures, and expected consequences to the appropriate individual, and has received a signed consent. Implied consent is common in an emergency situation when an ill or injured person is unable to grant actual consent. Implied consent allows paramedics and emergency medical technicians (EMT) to transport an individual to a health care facility to be treated in an emergency situation without the patient's written consent. A situation would generally be considered an emergency when a patient is suffering from a life-threatening disease or injury that requires immediate treatment.[12] Implied consent is also applied in an emergency situation when a minor child requires medical treatment and a parent's consent cannot be obtained.

Guardianship

The purpose of guardianship is to promote the general welfare of individuals who are incapacitated. Guardianship is a legal relationship, appointed by the court, between one individual (the guardian) and an incapacitated party. The guardian has the duty and the right to act on behalf of the incapacitated party to make decisions regarding the incapacitated person's life. Unless the guardian is limited by the court in his/her duties, management of all the personal, legal, and financial affairs of the incapacitated person is expected.

In general, guardianship is classified in two categories known as guardianship of person and guardianship of trust. Establishing guardianship is a means of establishing a legal system that provides incapacitated persons with the following rights:

- to participate as fully as possible in all decisions that affect them;
- to achieve essential and ongoing physical health and safety;
- to manage their financial resources;
- to develop or regain their abilities to the maximum extent possible;
- to accomplish the aforementioned objectives in the least restrictive environment and through the least restrictive alternatives.[13]

The appointed guardian can be a family member, such as a spouse or parent. When a family member is appointed it is often the next-of-kin. When a family member or next-of-kin is not able or willing to serve as guardian, or when the court determines that a family member is not the best choice for an incapacitated person, the appointed guardian can also be a professional guardian known to the court and trained in guardianship.

A Guardian Ad Litem is a guardian appointed to represent a child. This is necessary when there is a conflict between the parent(s) and the injured child or when there is no one who can adequately represent the best interests of the child. This can occur in child abuse cases or in other estranged domestic proceedings, such as custody and visitation proceedings. This also occurs when the parents are deceased or incapacitated. The Guardian Ad Litem has a duty to legally advocate for the child's best interests, which may include access to appropriate health care, special education, and/or even legal defense in the case of an accident. Sometimes the Guardian Ad Litem is an attorney appointed by the court, or can be the next-of-kin, or a professional guardian.

MALPRACTICE

Malpractice is professional negligence that refers to any misconduct or lack of skills in carrying out professional responsibilities. For malpractice to exist, negligence must be proven, and the four elements of negligence must be present: duty, breach of duty, causation, and injury.

1. Duty owed means that the provider has a responsibility to make reasonable decisions. In terms of a case manager, the reasonable decision may center around whether an appropriate referral for services or products was made.
2. Breach of Duty means that the duty was breached by an action or inaction.
3. Causation means that there is a definitive connection between the breach by action, or inaction, and the damage that resulted.
4. Injury means that damages to the patient resulted from the occurrence of the first three elements.

Malpractice and negligence are *unintentional torts*, meaning that harm was not intended at the time of the occurrence. Intentional torts are those wrongful acts carried out with intent to harm, such as assault, battery, invasion of privacy, and slander. A tort law is a law that addresses a wrongful act, whether intentional or unintentional, against a person or property. The most common law affecting health care practice is that of torts.

The incidence of patients claiming malpractice on the part of health care professionals has, unfortunately, increased over the past several years. Physicians are particularly vulnerable to malpractice claims because they are the health care professionals with ultimate responsibility for the care of the patient. However, case managers can also be held legally liable in a malpractice lawsuit. For this reason, all case managers should investigate obtaining professional liability insurance. Organizations like the American Nurses Association (ANA) and the Case Management Society of America (CMSA) offer group rates for liability insurance that are affordable by most professionals. Professional liability insurance will protect case managers in their own actions or inactions while performing the role of case management.

CONFIDENTIALITY

Confidentiality is a key issue in the discussions of today's health care system. Protecting patient confidentiality respects the patient's right to self-determination. As a health care professional, the case manager is ethically bound to maintain the maximum amount of confidentiality possible in matters of health and finances on behalf of the patient. Case managers may struggle with the knowledge that a patient continues to abuse his or her own health, such as refusing to complete a personal PT regime critical to recovery, or refusing to take daily HAART medication for the management of AIDs. Does it become the job of the case manager to become a watchdog—to judge or even deny services to the patient? This is an ethical issue of confidentiality that each case manager will undoubtedly face from time to time, and will need to come to terms with as a professional working with the patient.

Confidentiality and the issues of confidentiality in health care are far-reaching, diverse, and complex. Confidentiality is protected by federal law under HIPAA (see chapter eight) and under accreditation mandates by the Joint Commission on Accreditation of Healthcare Organizations (JCAHO). In 1988, JCAHO identified privacy and confidentiality as two patient rights. Further, many case managers are governed ethically to maintain patient confidentiality through their individual licensures and practice acts. The ANA's *Standards of Clinical Nursing Practice* require the nurse to maintain client confidentiality.

Rather than provide clear-cut answers about how and when to divulge information, these authorities can sometimes cause greater confusion for the case manager. In the collaborative role, the case manager is responsible to discuss a patient's condition, prognosis, and other confidential information with many different health care professionals and players—physicians, nurses, therapists, social services representatives, insurance company UR nurses and case managers, medical coding and billing personnel, risk managers and quality improvement professionals, claims adjusters, attorneys, and the patient's family or caregiver. In view of the many restrictions placed on confidentiality, it is a good rule of thumb for the case manager to reveal and discuss only the information that is essential for the other party to know—that which is in the best interests of the patient.

Special circumstances, diagnoses, and conditions are governed under various states' legislation that further convolute the rules regarding patient confidentiality. Examples include medical records of patients seeking treatment in drug and alcohol abuse rehabilitation programs, and records of HIV-positive patients. Most states have some degree of confidentiality for individuals with HIV-positive test results, including mandates for disclosure of HIV information, and for obtaining consents for testing procedures.

Patient Security

Despite large variation in state laws, one of the common challenges faced by all health care professionals is how to document, file, store, and share medical data in a way that promotes quality, timely health care for the patient, while still ensuring patient confidentiality and security of personal medical information. By far the most comprehensive legislation mandating confidentiality and patient security is HIPAA. HIPAA's relationship with patient security is discussed in detail in Chapter eight.

HIPPA re-engineers how health care professionals have traditionally viewed patient security. The Act requires full disclosure to a patient, upon request, of all entities who have obtained information unrelated to the patient's treatments, or payment of treatments. This information must be provided to the patient within 60 days of his/her request. Further, health care entities can no longer require patients to sign release forms authorizing release of medical information, as a condition of treating the patient. Before information on the patient is transferred to another entity, the entity possessing the information must receive a written advance consent from the patient. The significant point of this is that a single consent signature can no longer be used. Rather, additional signatures will be needed for many types of disclosures, such as a case manager's release of information to an employer in a workers' compensation case.

There are many key provisions of the HIPAA regulations as defined in Chapter eight. Complete information on patient security issues promulgated by HIPAA can be accessed on the U.S. Department of Health and Human Services Website at www.hhs.gov.

CONFLICT OF INTEREST

A conflict of interest can be described as a situation in which a person has a private or a personal interest sufficient to appear to influence the objective exercise of his or her official duties.[14] When the private interest comes into conflict with the official duty of the individual, the conflict can potentially interfere with objective professional judgment. Conflict of interest can be apparent and potential as well as actual. In an apparent conflict of interest, a reasonable person can believe that the professional's judgment is likely to be compromised. A potential conflict of interest is one that may develop into an actual conflict of interest, and an actual conflict of interest is when the conflict does occur.

In the role of the case manager, there are many opportunities to unintentionally engage in apparent, potential, or actual conflict of interest. The following are just a few examples of conflict of interest:

- You work as a case manager in an acute care hospital where a manufacturing representative for glucose monitors visits often to introduce you and other staff members to equipment available for your patients. Although you do not directly purchase the equipment, the rep recognizes your ability to educate and influence patients' decisions about equipment. Because of your acquaintance with the rep, you are able to secure a summer job for your daughter with the rep's company.
- You use the computer software licensed to your employer for your own private consulting work by copying the software and placing it on your personal computer.
- You work for an insurance company that has many home health care agencies on its list of providers. You accept a substantial gift from one of the home health agencies at Christmas or Hanukkah, which happens to be the agency you commonly refer for your patients

Obviously, conflict of interest can and does occur often in health care. In order to avoid conflict of interest, the case manager should continuously consider whether the situation is likely to interfere, or appear to interfere with independent, objective judgment. If this is not clear, consider whether trust would be compromised if other people knew of the situation. There are multiple ways to manage conflict of interest. One is to avoid the conflict altogether. Another is to disclose the perceived, potential or actual conflict of interest to the appropriate parties before participating in the action. Another is to abstain from any decision-making surrounding the private interest.

Usually, it is easier to recognize conflict of interest in someone else than it is to recognize it in oneself. Personal interests cloud objectivity, or the individual may believe he/she can always separate private interest from the official duty, thus failing to critically analyze potential conflict of interest before it arises. A good practice is to follow the following metaphor:

Pass the situation into your mind, where you analyze it, and out of your heart, where you feel it. If it still seems right, it probably is.

ACCESS TO CARE

The final section to be discussed in this chapter on legal and ethical issues is access to care. Access to care pertains to the ability or inability of individuals to obtain necessary health care services and products due to economics, location, culture, or other innate factors. For example, The Henry J. Kaiser Family Foundation reports on its website (www.kff.org) that immigrants account for 20 percent of America's uninsured. Kaiser cites the welfare reform law of 1996 as having significant impact on the number of immigrants who are uninsured, because the law restricts Medicaid eligibility for certain immigrant populations. This is an example of how culture, economics, and legislation all impact access to care.

Patients' access to health care is a growing legal and ethical dilemma amidst a growing population of uninsured Americans. There are more than 43 million Americans without health insurance in this country, according to the Physicians' Work Group on Universal Coverage. The Physicians' Work Group is a coalition that includes the American Academy of Family Physicians, American Academy of Pediatrics, American College of Emergency Physicians, American College of Obstetricians and Gynecologists, American College of Physicians, American Society of Internal Medicine, American College of Surgeons, and the American Medical Association. This coalition raises awareness and concern regarding access to care for patients, and estimates that more than 47 million Americans will be uninsured by 2005.[15]

The U.S. Agency for Healthcare Research and Quality (AHRQ) has completed significant research on access to care in the U.S. In 2000, the agency released results of a study that shows Asians and Pacific Islanders on the West Coast had worse access to care than whites or any other ethnic group.[16] This study is significant because it indicates that economics is not a factor in this group of uninsured Americans. Asians had the highest proportion of high-income people and a larger population of well-educated individuals than other groups in the study, factors that are usually associated with increased access to care. The study cited cultural differences as the innate factor contributing to poor access to care.

Barriers to access care are diverse and far-reaching. Despite the fact that laws can contribute to existing barriers, legal and ethical circumstances may also assist patients in receiving access to care. As noted in Chapter eight, EMTALA is federal legislation guaranteeing a person's right to emergency medical care. HIPAA protects an employee from losing group health insurance coverage if the employee changes jobs. From an ethical standpoint, Chapter two cites how case managers have a responsibility to provide services for an individual, regardless of an ability to pay.

Access issues can also pertain to patients who are insured. Access may be limited or denied to care such as preventive services, routine care, specialty services, and/or health care education due to the type of insurance policy carried by the patient. Access to care can also be limited or denied to individuals who have insurance coverage, but limited or denied care can occur because of inadequacies in the health care delivery system or in the health insurance system. Examples include delays in receiving approval for services; waiting time before appointments with primary care physicians or specialists; accessing a staff person on the telephone to ask questions; and not obtaining diagnostic testing results in a timely manner. Despite the situation and whether services will be paid, case managers have an ethical responsibility to provide whatever services are possible that are in the best interests of the patient. This is why resource management is such an important part of the process of case management (see Chapter five). Resource management can provide potential solutions when access to care is limited or when barriers to care exist.

Sometimes access to care will not be achieved because the patient refuses the care that is available or offered. This situation is especially frustrating for the case manager accustomed to working diligently to access appropriate services. However, a patient's right to self-determination dictates that the patient can refuse access to available care. Before accepting a patient's refusal of care, the case manager should ensure that the patient has received adequate information to make an informed decision. If a patient has received adequate information, is able to make an informed decision, and still refuses care, the case manager should document this activity, including the information about the expected outcomes both with and without the service, and that the patient has refused the service.

REFERENCES

1, 3. Banja,J. Hitting the mark: Ethics in case management. *Continuing Care*.1997: 24,5:29–45.

2. Taylor, C. Transforming the culture of care: a non-elective mission of moral integrity. *CMSA 10th Annual Case Management Conference Proceedings Manual*. Little Rock, AR. CMSA. 2000:464–473.

4. Case Management Society of America. *Standards of practice for case management*. Little Rock, AR. CMSA. 1995:22–23.

5. Tillman, V. Ethics. In Howe, R, ed. *Case management for healthcare professionals*. Chicago, IL. Precept Press; 1994:35–38.

6. Peplau, H. Is healthcare a right? *Image: Journal of Nursing Scholarship*. 1974: 7,1:4–10.

7. Powell, S. *Nursing case management*. Philadelphia, PA. Lippincott. 1996:4,2:155–156.

8. Mantel, D.L. Laws on death and dying. *Advance for Nurses*. 2001: 2,2:17– 38.

9. Do doctors undertreat dying elderly or overtreat those dying young? *Medical Interface*. 1996: 3,4:43.

10. Mitchell, E.R. Elder abuse basics part 5: What is abandonment? Available at: http://socialwork.about.com.

11. Child abuse and neglect state statutes elements. *National Clearinghouse on Child Abuse and Neglect Information*. U.S. Department of Health and Human Services, Administration for Children and Families. Washington, D.C.: U.S. Government Printing Office; 1999:1.

12, 13. Romano, J. *Legal rights of the catastrophically ill and injured: a family guide*. Philadelphia, PA. Rosenstein & Romano;1996: 24–26.

14. McDonald, M. Ethics and conflict of interest. *Centre for Applied Ethics Website*. Available at: www.ethics.ubc.ca.

15. Eaton, J.A. Coalition urges renewed focus on uninsured. *Physicians Financial News*. 1999: 17,12:1–22.

16. Snyder, R.E., Cunningham, W. et al. Access to medical care reported by Asians and Pacific Islanders in a West Coast physician group association. *Medical Care Research and Review*. 2000: 57,2:196–215.

EMERGING ISSUES 11

The best is saved for last! This chapter transports the reader into the year 2030, where case managers can examine trends that just three short decades ago were being pioneered. Today, these trends have paved the way for a new fantasy—or ones that have yet to be envisioned. Consumers of healthcare services have analytical sophistication stemming from personal familiarity with information technologies. They are consumers of comparison-shopping, and as a result have transformed major industries to meet their diverse wellness and living needs.

Interstellar travel, control of inherent human healing power, cognition-enhancing drugs, beneficial uses of low level radiation, and new sources of energy that faced skepticism at the turn of the 21st century are now accepted realities. The world population has reached the peak predicted in terms of aging, with 1.5 billion people over the age of 60 worldwide. The world has seen many positive results of health promotion that have been stressed since the turn of the century.[1]

One of the major industries that has prospered from technological advances is the health care industry. The health care system now embraces a much broader definition of health and wellness than it did in the past. Health and wellness are viewed not just as the absence of disease. Rather, to be healthy and well means to be physically, emotionally, mentally, and spiritually whole despite the presence of chronic disease.[2] Consumers of health care services appreciate a core paradox of health care: that to healthfully embrace life, one must accept eventual death. In this regard, one sees not only health, but also disease as an opportunity for growth…even a gift. Health and wellness allow life to be well lived and death to occur with dignity.[3]

Contrary to earlier practices, the center of the health care system is not the doctor, the hospital CEO, the insurance company, government, or the employer, but the individual. This concept comes from the belief that it is individual life that matters most, so it is up to the individual to set his/her course for improving quality of life. In this patient-centered, choice-based system, health care professionals play a vital yet secondary and facilitative role, providing expertise, easy access to information, and therapeutic assistance when requested.

Today, high-touch has merged with high-tech. Brain surgery is preceded by massage and prayer, and followed by homeopathy and music therapy. In the event of an illness, multidisciplinary teams are mobilized to care for the patient, and families are invited to join them. Professional caregivers are peer-approved and experienced at collaborating as a team, recognizing the strengths and limitations in each individual specialty. Since a strong emphasis continues to be placed on prevention, personal responsibility, and simple complementary procedures, such as acupuncture and other technologic advances, chronic illness is treated proactively. Thus, health care costs continue to decline even with the ever-aging population.

Today, malpractice suits are rare, since health care delivery is a perfected science and art, blending the best of both paradigms. Employers offer financial incentives to employees who demonstrate healthy behaviors. Access to affordable, appropriate health care is universal and considered a fundamental human right. These changes have resulted from the new way society views the community. If someone in the family is sick, the community mobilizes resources to assist that person. This has resulted in a decrease in costs of absenteeism and lost productively to employers. Subsequently, opportunities for healing practices are available in the home, at work, and through community centers. Further, the acceptance of death has made advance directives commonplace and the dying process dignified.

Health care in 2030 is viewed as a global business that allows advances and practices to be shared in order to improve health status and the quality of life of all people. The next section will look at how multiculturalism has been accepted and used to enhance health and wellness in a dynamic health care environment.

MULTI-CULTURAL ISSUES AND HEALTH BEHAVIOR

Today, due to globalization, nations are able to assist each other to improve health and welfare for all. Just 30 years ago, at the turn of the century, globalization caused uncertainty and fear among many people. Now, consumers are witnesses to the benefits that have allowed interdependence throughout the world. As health promoters, clinicians recognize the power of linking global values with local action. Through encouragement of global solidarity while nurturing diversity, clinicians have helped to shape events in line with the values of human equity and fairness for all, regardless of culture.[4]

More and more governments are recognizing good health as a critical element of human security. In some nations this foresight has become the basis of foreign policy. An example of this is seen in the cooperation that the United Nations has provided to Africa as they address issues related to HIV/AIDS. As the U.S. eradicated polio in the last century, so now Africa has been empowered with pharmaceutical resources to implement a massive inoculation campaign to eradicate this once-feared disease.

Sustained improvement in International Health has also been a key theme in the Millennium Report by the United Nation's Security-General.[5] Major elements have been recognized on a global level. People need to possess the power to improve their own health through knowledge, to be in a position to choose better health, and the empowerment to make decisions and stick to them. For health promoters to assist in this goal, a philosophy has been accepted that has allowed issues of multiculturalism to be better understood. If one discriminates against people of color, he/she loses access to the richness of many cultures. By practicing respect for an individual's health practices, faith beliefs, traditions, and cultural orientation, that respect is returned to health care professionals.[6]

E-HEALTH

Information technology is a powerful mechanism of change that has accelerated economic development, augmented health care services through telemedicine, and increased the world's ability to share information. The Internet, as a method for consumers to access information, was already becoming the tool to educate and empower people around the world at the turn of the century. The Internet has accelerated a form of personal communication that allows society to be self-sufficient and equipped to self-manage their health care decisions.

Consumers today know more and demand more from providers than ever before in the history of this country. Those with chronic diseases are now able to stay current with new advances that affect their individual conditions. For example, a patient with amyotrophic lateral sclerosis is able to access up-to-date information regarding new drugs and treatments that have shown success in reducing complications of ALS. It is only a matter of time before this neuromuscular disease joins muscular dystrophy and multiple sclerosis in being eradicated.

Consumers are able to download information for a small USPS fee and email it directly to their physician, so that a discussion on the efficacy of that treatment can be discussed online between both parties during the physician's regular Internet visiting hours. By taking advantage of this common technology, consumers take an active role in all aspects of their health care decisions.

The pharmaceutical industry has seen the impact and has adapted their products and services to both providers and consumers. The Internet allows consumers to use their browsers to compare prices of similar drugs, and to use their Medical Savings Accounts to opt for higher-priced drugs that their insurance plans will not cover or include on the formulary. This shift has been significant for the industry where brand and generic drugs compete for the market share. To compete, suppliers of brand drugs are forced to offer supplementary services to justify higher prices. Online disease management programs and online talking pharmacies that offer personalized advice regarding specific effects of medications have been a benefit to consumers.[7]

Another trend that has resulted from E-health is that, globally, consumers are digging deeper into their pockets to fund their health care needs. As a result, the way health care systems deliver care has changed to better accommodate this trend. Patient satisfaction is critically important and is quantified through consistent survey techniques. What has been learned through these surveys is that the major drivers for patient satisfaction are the patient encounter, scheduling, and transparency of the care process.[8]

TELEHEALTH

Telehealth has been an accepted practice, especially in rural acute centers, for more than a decade. A robot assists an orthopedic surgeon to drill the precise cavity for a hip replacement; a neurosurgery student physician in Spain is able to perform a new procedure that has been perfected in the U.S. by using a virtual reality (VR) headpiece. The VR headpiece allows him to view the specific parts of the procedure as he operates. A busy cardiologist is able to closely monitor a 78-year-old patient at home through a wireless wristwatch that sends her vital signs to the physician's palm pilot. These technologies allow health care to be mobile, flexible, and meet demands to provide quality health care at a lower cost.

Another example is seen in the use of real-time biosensors that are used to read and transmit responses to physical and chemical changes. Patients with diabetes use these sensors, equipped with electrodes and immobilized enzymes, to continuously monitor glucose levels. This eliminates the archaic and invasive need for fingersticks and blood draws so common at the turn of the century. Normalized glucose levels are maintained by controlling insulin from an implantable pump that delivers precise doses in micrometers as needed.[9] This practice has eradicated diabetic comas.

Today, health care providers are using electronic data to more efficiently use diagnostic tools, surgical procedures, and to assess patients more precisely. Diseases are being treated proactively with applied therapeutic interventions across all settings. The computer and robotics have revolutionized the way surgical procedures are performed. Robots provide decision support before surgery, facilitate less-invasive surgery, provide surgical tools customized to the patient, and help guide the surgeon's hand during a procedure. This, along with imaging devices, has allowed the surgeon to have full-range eye movement in the operative surroundings while, at the same time, view 3D images of internal body parts. Surgery is now much more precise, with fewer complications and extraordinarily enhanced outcomes.[10] This is evident in cardiac bypass surgery, which was requiring short-stay hospitalizations during the turn of the century, but now can be performed in the comfort of the physician's office.

Still, the home is considered the center for health care delivery. Since the advent of the ability of electric companies to run communication services over standard electric power lines, high-speed, low-cost access to the Internet and other communication services are now in all homes and businesses. This access allows for sound, voice, and data communication channels that provide for sophisticated telehealth and telemedicine applications to be incorporated to facilitate communication among the patient, the family, and health care providers. Outcomes have resulted in allowing health care providers from remote sites to help consumers to care for their family members in the home. This access has also decreased caregiver stress because of personalized support readily available through the health care team.

AGING POPULATION

Information gained from research that focuses on the special physical and emotional needs of older persons provides the world with a better understanding of the unique aspects of aging. Older age is a distinct and unique phase of life in which a person's senses; hearing, seeing, taste, and touch, along with physical strength, mobility, and dexterity undergo significant changes. These alterations in a person's physical abilities need not be seen as disabilities, given the advances and availability that technology and environmental design have made over time.[11] By employing state-of-the-art information and appropriate design products and materials, adaptations to the home and the workplace are commonly performed and provide ways for people to compensate the changes occurring during the normal aging process. These advances have allowed people to truly age-in-place and to achieve freedom of movement, safety, and to remain involved in life's events.

Due to globalization, we realize that people are basically the same everywhere in the world and that everyone is living longer. Each country is dealing with the graying of their population in its own way. Progressive countries are ensuring that older persons are well integrated into society as significant contributors, based on their life experiences and acquired wisdom. Statistics show that, every month, one million people in the world turn 60.[12]

The Western models of separation between age groups have been found to no longer be a viable option. When older people are separated into communities, their health deteriorates, placing a physical as well as an economic burden on the health care system and family. Conversely, when older persons are actively integrated into community life, they stay healthier and life becomes more enjoyable, productive, and satisfying. This is important, considering that most people retire at age 80, so that a normal life expectancy of 20–30 years after retirement remains. It is important, therefore, that people stay as healthy and as functional as possible so that they may experience the active retirement they planned.

GENETICS AND BIOTECHNOLOGY

The 21st century has been called the Biotech Century. Tremendous advances have been made as a result of this technology in predicting risk and in the development of aggressive treatments and products. Biotechnology allows society to better manage several forms of chronic disease, such as cardiovascular disease, kidney disease, cancer, and diseases of the blood. These advances enable scientists to prepare practitioners in technology who can either add to or correct genes that cause specific diseases in the human body, in many cases eradicating or significantly slowing disease processes. In addition, researchers have developed small-molecule therapeutics that regulate the function of a number of different complex, multi-genetic diseases and therapies, such as arthritis, wound healing, and immune-deficiencies. Slower to develop have been gene-based treatment for mental illness, but the progress that has been made enables practitioners to better diagnose and manage mental diseases more effectively. Another breakthrough that is part of this success is the ability to proactively treat birth defects in utero with gene therapy.[13]

Interestingly, the space agency NASA, a leader in space technology, is able to mimic processes in the biological world. Probes are sent into space that have life-like properties. They are robust, self-reliant, adaptable, and evolvable. They can self-heal when damaged, and have complete self-awareness. They are able to respond to hostile human conditions that they find on distant planets. The plan, according to the current NASA administrator, is to put colonies of robots on planets to thrive, move about, and to mimic human characteristics, such as to manipulate objects with the dexterity of a human hand, explore large areas, and have psychological attributes that allow them to express emotions, and have the ability to select and remove leaders in order to perform tasks. The goal of this work is to provide leadership to the developing biotech industry as it relates to our mission in space, and ultimately bring back benefits to earth, to create biologically inspired products that will dramatically improve the quality of life on earth.[14]

GLOBAL CASE MANAGEMENT/CARE COORDINATORS

Care coordinators (CCs) today maintain the essence of the practice of case management established in the early 20th century, and fine-tuned at the start of the 21st century. They are primarily known as accelerators of health care. They are able to adapt to present health care environments, using various disciplines and professionals. Their standards of practice have evolved to be standards to which all care managers adhere, regardless of discipline or license.

The role of CCs remains dynamic. They are primarily used to bridge the gap that technology has created. CCs assist consumers to better understand how to access information, to use sophisticated home-based technology that has evolved over time, and to be intermediaries to handle health care needs when called upon in crises.

Unlike case management practice at the turn of the century, today's CCs are financed directly by consumers and/or employers. They directly fund CC services to ensure that they are receiving the best care to address complicated conditions. The major impact of this practice was felt by general practitioners, who previously had assumed the role of gatekeepers of care but now are responsible solely for diagnosing and prescribing treatment. CCs are intermediaries who function at different levels and with different specializations according to the needs of their clients. Some consumers may demand human contact or may wish to contract with CCs through virtual agents who provide the service of sorting through health information to meet a particular profile.[15]

All CCs are prepared in advanced practice and have a vast level of expertise in the health care industry and from other health disciplines. Unlike their counterpart case managers at the turn of the century, all CCs must achieve certification to practice. Professionals wishing to enter the field are mentored until they are comfortable in their role as determined by competency evaluations.

Returning to the present, readers can see that the information presented throughout this book sets the groundwork for today's case managers, as well as tomorrow's care coordinators or case managers. It is unknown what the practice of case management will be called in 30 years, but it is assumed that case management must remain flexible and dynamic to adapt to changes that the future will bring. To enhance the viability of the practice, case managers need to take an active role in sharing their expertise and knowledge as mentors. Case managers, in collaboration with other health care professionals throughout the care continuum, must ensure that the changes they create deliver the promises they claim. The goal is to provide quality, cost-effective care, in the least restrictive setting, at the most appropriate time. This is one concept that has not changed, nor will not change, over time, but will continue to drive the quest for excellence.

In closing, the authors want to thank you for sharing your time reading the pages of this book. We hope the book will serve as a valuable tool to improve your practice, and to provide structure as you learn more about case management or prepare for certification. We hope we have truly clarified the process and essence of case management, and have fortified you with information to produce best practices in your individual settings. We hope that you have enjoyed the ride!

REFERENCES

1, 11, 12. Russell, B. Toward a society for all ages. Available at: http://www.isdesignet.com/Magazine/Mar'99/cover.html

2, 3. Vision 2020 a positive future for healthcare. Available at: www.integrativemedalliance.org .

4, 5. Brundtland, G. Fifth global conference on health promotion. Available at: www.who.int

6. Acosta, B. & Higgins, D. Corondelet/Santa Cruz parish nurse program. In. Cohen, E., De Back, V. *The Outcomes Mandate, Case Management in Health Care Today*. St. Louis, MO. Mosby: 1999:132–137.

7. Industry Solutions. Gateway to the future of healthcare. Available at: www.microsoft.com/europe/industry/healthcare/features/1817.htm.

8, 15. Price Waterhouse Coopers. HealthCast 2010: Smaller world, bigger expectations. Available at: http://www.pwchealth.com/ healthcast2010.html

9, 10. Marietti, C. Advanced medical techniques and technologies are on their way to a facility near you. *Healthcare Informatics*. 1998: 23,4:38–47

13, 14. Anderson, W. Eight visions of the future: Biotech 2030. Available at: http://www.biospace.com/articles/010600_print.cfm

Additional Available Manuals Authored
by Kathleen Moreo and Anne Llewellyn:

Disability management specialists and rehabilitation specialists will gain diverse knowledge in the "Disability Management and Rehabilitation Specialist's Handbook" (2003). This spiral-bound book of more than 100 pages is designed to assist the CDMS applicant in taking the CDMS examination. It is also an excellent resource guide for all healthcare professionals working in rehabilitation case management, workers' compensation, disability management, vocational counseling and other related specialty areas in healthcare rehabilitation.

Occupational Therapists, Life Care Planners, Assistive Technology Specialists, Home Modification Experts, Contractors, Architects, Engineers and public health nurses have testified to the value of "Understanding Environmental Access" (2003). This spiral-bound book of more than 100 pages is designed to provide cutting edge information in a first-ever compilation of the techniques, principles, standards, and practices constituting environmental access. This manual also serves to embrace the core body of knowledge constituting an environmental access specialist, having been authored following five years of study of the essential elements of U.S.-based home modifications, universal access, ADA-compliance, and barrier free design. It is also an excellent resource guide for all healthcare and environmental access professionals assisting the disabled and elderly in achieving environmental access, whether in workers' compensation, disability management, life care planning, vocational rehabilitation, grant administration, Medicaid waiver, or direct-to-consumer venues.

"The Essentials of Case Management: Tools, Techniques, Principles and Practices" manual has been successfully used since 1995 by case managers who are stepping up to certification; by health care practitioners entering the field of case management; by seasoned case managers wishing to learn the how-to's of CM in a different pay system and setting from their own; and by professors in the academic setting. is a 300 page manual used by thousands of case managers since 1995 to assist them in understanding and identifying the core components and essential elements of case management. It is the official course manual used in PRIME's onsite 1- and 2-day Essentials of Case Management program, and the basis of PRIME's 17-hour online program. The book carries literally hundreds of testimonials on file pertaining to its usefulness. *The Essentials of Case Management: Tools, Techniques, Principles and Practices* **is now only available as a 17-hour CE online course at www.primeinc.org and was updated in December 2004.**

All these books are available for purchase via credit cards on PRIME's website at www.primeinc.org

APPENDIX A

REVIEW QUESTIONS

1. Tools that can be utilized to identify patients who may benefit from a disease management program include all **EXCEPT**:
   a. ICD-9 codes.
   b. CPT codes.
   c. utilization data.
   d. radiology data.

2. Which is **NOT** included as one of the three major elements that are globally accepted to achieve health and wellness?
   a. knowledge.
   b. to be in a position to choose better health.
   c. the empowerment to make decisions and stick to those decisions.
   d. money.

3. If a case manager is working with a home care agency within a managed care network and there is a complaint regarding the quality of the staff they are sending, the case manager should first address this complaint with the:
   a. accrediting agency that oversees the managed care network.
   b. quality department within the managed care organization.
   c. home care agency's director of nursing.
   d. risk management department within the managed care organization.

4. Social service agencies may differ from volunteer organizations because:
   a. they usually require the patient to meet certain eligibility criteria not required by most voluntary organizations.
   b. they charge fees, while volunteer organizations are free.
   c. social service agencies are financed with state funds, while volunteer organizations are financed with federal funds.
   d. volunteer organizations are more loosely structured with all-volunteer staffs

5. Which health assessment screening tool would be a common choice when assessing the chronic alcoholic patient?
   a. ROSE.
   b. SF 36.
   c. BASIS 32.
   d. OASIS.

6. The 80/20 rule demonstrates:
   a. that there is a direct ratio between health care spending and the at risk population that uses health care resources.

b. that supervisors have a way to determine case management caseloads.

c. the ratio between the insured and the uninsured.

d. the ratio of those covered by private insurance and those covered by managed care organizations.

7. A mother of an adolescent diabetic calls the diabetic case manager to seek assistance for her son, who has missed school due to sluggishness and oversleeping. During the conversation, the mother informs the case manager that her son is not sticking to the diet and has had high sugar levels over the past week. The case manager uses what skill(s) to address this problem of noncompliance?

a. negotiation.

b. conflict resolution and problem solving.

c. consultation.

d. accountability.

8. The case manager working in the provider setting whose role is to ensure that resources are used in an appropriate manner for the payer and the provider may be found in which setting?

a. Hospital.

b. Managed care organization.

c. Professional organization.

d. Credentialing organization.

9. In a stated contract used by the provider delivering services, it is implied that:

a. costs will be competitive.

b. quality will be assured.

c. confidentiality will be maintained.

d. the provider will be paid for services rendered

10. The first phase of the case management process is:

a. patient identification and referral.

b. examination of the benefits and limitations.

c. assessment of the patient.

d. development of a treatment plan.

11. Dietary planning is an essential part of the diabetic patient's regimen. The American Diabetes Association recommends which of the following caloric guidelines for daily meal planning?

a. 50% complex carbohydrate; 20%–25% protein; 20%–25% fat.

b. 45% complex carbohydrate; 25%–30% protein; 30%–35% fat.

c. 70% complex carbohydrate; 20%–30% protein; 10%–20% fat.

d. 60% complex carbohydrate; 12%–15% protein; 20%–25% fat.

12. The ultimate goal of a comprehensive rehabilitation program is to:

a. decrease the services needed for appropriate patient management.

b. reduce the physical, emotional, and economic effects of a disability on the injured or ill individual.

c. limit the long-term costs of services for the client.

d. maximize the available services to enhance the treatment plan.

13. The primary reason to conduct a job analysis is to:

a. prevent further work injuries in the work place.

b. identify essential job functions necessary to perform the job.

c. determine the educational requirements necessary to perform the job.

d. determine the job market in a given demographic area.

14. To prevent carpal tunnel syndrome, a typist's wrists should be in which position?

a. Flexed.

b. Extended.

c. Neutral.

d. Comfortably at a 45-degree angle.

15. Efficient data management systems allow for data to be analyzed and evaluated as part of the:

 a. continuous quality improvement process.

 b. risk management process in malpractice cases.

 c. billing process in provider organizations.

 d. coding process in medical records.

16. By incorporating best practices, case managers achieve all of the following except:

 a. improved clinical outcomes.

 b. improved administrative efficiencies.

 c. reduced cost in healthcare.

 d. eliminate chronic illness due to best practices.

17. When a case manager is practicing family-centered case management, he/she is enabling the family. Enabling families means to:

 a. impart the medical coordination of care to appropriate family members.

 b. create opportunities for the family to become more competent and independent in meeting their needs.

 c. locate secondary providers to assist the family.

 d. complete a grievance process to the insurance company when services needed by the patient/ family are denied.

18. Screening tools can be effectively used to:

 a. screen patients who may be costly to the system because of the type of illness.

 b. assess patients' own perceptions and knowledge of their health status.

 c. provide the number of chronic illnesses and diseases in a managed care organization.

 d. identify patients with specific conditions who are at risk so that teaching can prevent hospital admissions.

19. When a case manager arranges equipment delivery to a patient's home, she/he should:

 a. be present in the home at the time of delivery to provide instructional use of the equipment to the patient and family or caregiver.

 b. disclose the cost of the equipment to the patient.

 c. be available to sign the delivery order.

 d. ensure that the patient or family or caregiver is provided with contact information on the equipment manufacturer, as well as the agency or company providing the equipment.

20. The approach used for resource management is a(n):

 a. goal oriented approach.

 b. demand management approach.

 c. evidence-based medicine approach.

 d. capitated funding approach.

21. In a viatical settlement, how much the insurance company will pay the viator is usually determined by the:

 a. determination by the life-care planner.

 b. viator's living will.

 c. amount negotiated by the viator.

 d. life expectancy of the viator.

22. When calling the managed care utilization management specialist to obtain authorization for an elective hysterectomy, the acute care case manager must provide what information?

 a. complete medical record detailing the patient's history of severe cramping and intensive bleeding episodes.

b. diagnostic testing that supports the need for the hysterectomy.
c. written order from the surgeon who will perform the procedure.
d. signed consent form showing that the patient has agreed to the procedure and understands the risks and benefits.

23. A physician has decided that a bone marrow transplant is the treatment of choice for 38-year-old woman with breast cancer. He receives a denial from the woman's HMO. He feels that he has the supporting documentation to justify the procedure. The next step that the physician should take to ensure that the patient receives medically appropriate care is to:
    a. file a quick-claim lawsuit against the HMO.
    b. send a letter to the state insurance commissioner's office protesting the decision.
    c. inform the patient that she should submit a grievance against the HMO.
    d. file an appeal with the HMO with supportive documentation that justifies the bone marrow transplant.

24. Outcomes that are anticipated from utilization management and case management are:
    a. an increase in the credentials of professional staff.
    b. better use of resources, containment of costs, and quality health care delivery.
    c. a decrease in health care costs from administrative overlap decrease.
    d. the creation of a new accreditation body to oversee the new model of care coordination.

25. Weight reduction programs that are geared to children strive to:
    a. encourage weight loss.
    b. point out poor eating habits.
    c. encourage parents to control the child's diet.
    d. boost self-esteem and communication skills.

26. The primary goal of disease monitoring is to:
    a. reduce the amount of calls that the treating physician receives due to complications arising in a chronically ill patient.
    b. make the patient aware of any changes that require hospitalization, and discern minor changes that can wait for a regular office visit with the treating physician.
    c. educate the patient to report all positive and negative changes, for more accurate monitoring.
    d. inform the patient that, if there are more than three admissions to the hospital, the patient will be dropped from the disease management program.

27. The symptoms of restrictive lung disease include all of the following **except:**
    a. reduction of air volume, capacity, and noncompliant lungs.
    b. narrowing of airways.
    c. inadequate oxygenation of hemoglobin.
    d. the ability to exhale a large tidal volume.

28. A living will designates:
    a. whether the patient's physician has the authority to make treatment decisions in the event the patient is unable to make medical decisions.
    b. whether an individual desires life-prolonging treatment in the event that he/she is unable to make medical decisions.
    c. whether advance directives are necessary.
    d. whether accelerated death benefits are available to the patient.

29. Title III of the Americans with Disabilities Act is federally enforced by the:
    a. Department of Justice.
    b. Equal Employment Opportunity Commission.

c. Architectural and Transportation Barriers Compliance Board.

d. Department of Federal Affairs.

30. The Health Insurance Portability and Accountability Act provides:

    a. opportunity for an employee to accept a new job and maintain his/her former group health insurance for 62 days maximum.

    b. capability for an employer to exclude a new employee from the group health plan if the employee has a significant medical history.

    c. capability for an employee to move to a new employer health plan without denial or exclusion of benefits if there is no break in group health coverage exceeding 62 days.

    d. opportunity for an employee to accept a new job and maintain his/her former group health insurance for 18 months.

31. The Family and Medical Leave Act of 1993 allows for:

    a. unpaid leave for up to 6 months for eligible employees.

    b. benefits received by an employee during illness to be treated as non-taxable income.

    c. paid leave for up to 16 weeks for eligible employees.

    d. unpaid leave for up to 12 weeks for eligible employees.

32. Subrogation is defined as:

    a. the legal process by which an insurance company seeks from a third party, who has caused a loss, recovery of the amount paid to the policyholder.

    b. the insurance process by which coordinated health care payments are made by two or more benefit plans simultaneously.

    c. the insurance process by which a health care beneficiary can receive out-of-benefit services if a cost-benefit analysis is designed.

    d. the legal process by which health plan beneficiaries can recapture out-of-pocket expenses from their primary insurance company.

33. An HMO's primary goal is to:

    a. limit choices in the treatment plan.

    b. enhance cost savings through limitation of benefits.

    c. limit the policy holder's selection of a primary care physician.

    d. enhance the quality of care through a coordinated network.

34. Under the "own occupation" (own occ) rule in disability insurance, a person can:

    a. file a claim of wage-loss disability based on an inability to perform all aspects of the person's job.

    b. file a claim of wage-loss disability based on an inability to perform any one aspect of the person's job.

    c. rewrite his/her own job description to modify aspects of the job he/she cannot perform.

    d. sue the employer for the right to return to his/her own occupation.

35. Protecting patient confidentiality respects the patient's right to:

    a. self-esteem.

    b. self-determination.

    c. self-defense.

    d. self-incrimination.

36. There are two basic categories of guardianship. Guardianship of:

    a. person and guardianship of health.

    b. person and guardianship of estate.

    c. health and guardianship of property.

    d. person and guardianship of trusts.

37. A legal informed consent must include a competent person of legal age to consent; appropriate information given to and understood by the person consenting; and:
    a. written documentation of the intended treatment provided to the person consenting.
    b. a timeline of when the treatment is expected to occur.
    c. written or verbal information on what the outcome will be.
    d. freedom of choice by the person consenting.

38. By using sophisticated analytical tools, consumers of health care services will be able to:
    a. stay within their managed care network.
    b. do comparison shopping to ensure that products and services are of high quality and cost-effective to meet individual health care needs.
    c. use the Internet only to obtain products and services that are recommended by the treating physician.
    d. manage their own health care with no assistance from a health care professional.

39. As a result of the impact that E-health has had, the pharmaceutical industry has had to:
    a. step-up advertising efforts to the public, since they make the final choices.
    b. control advertisement efforts to the public, since the public is not trained to make health care decisions.
    c. offer online disease management programs and online pharmacy services to assist consumers to understand pharmaceutical choices.
    d. provide a way for physicians to be notified when a patient goes online to check out alternative services that they did not recommend.

40. The 21st century is known as the:
    a. biotech century.
    b. technologic century.
    c. century devoted to improving care to the elderly.
    d. century responsible for reforming the health care industry.

41. Clinical guidelines should be based on:
    a. patient request.
    b. clinical information.
    c. best practices.
    d. benchmarks

42. The life-care plan is a comprehensive written document that determines required medical, financial, psychological, spiritual, and social needs of an ill or injured person estimated over the:
    a. expected rehabilitation period.
    b. acute phase of the occupational illness or injury.
    c. acute injury or illness and up to 24 months after the injury/illness.
    d. person's lifetime.

43. To avoid stress or burnout, case managers performing ongoing resource management need to see themselves as:
    a. the decision makers regarding health care benefits.
    b. the center of the rehabilitation process.
    c. respected by the physician.
    d. successful in helping patients achieve progress.

44. The approach used for resource management is a(n):
    a. goal oriented approach.
    b. demand management approach.

c. evidence-based medicine approach.

d. capitated funding approach.

45. Which legislative act established vocational rehabilitation as a permanent federal program in 1935?

a. Vocational Rehabilitation and Training Act.

b. Social Security Disability Income Act.

c. Social Security Act.

d. Smith-Hughes Act.

46. The Rehabilitation Act of 1973 addresses:

a. public access requirements for all retail businesses.

b. required access for all forms of public transportation.

c. rights of disabled individuals to receive rehabilitation treatment, regardless of their ability to pay.

d. civil rights for all persons with disabilities.

47. In the past fee-for-service environment, health care services were:

a. reactive oriented—based on injury and illness needs.

b. wellness oriented—based on preventive maintenance.

c. economically oriented—based on capitated costs.

d. patient oriented—based on advocacy.

48. When an injured worker is receiving workers' compensation benefits, Medicare benefits are:

a. primary to workers' compensation benefits.

b. not applicable.

c. secondary to workers' compensation benefits.

d. reduced in accordance with the Resource Based Relative Value Scale.

49. Advance directives are also known as:

a. accelerated death benefits.

b. living wills.

c. the Patient Self-Determination Act.

d. viatical settlements.

50. Reporting of abuse is:

a. mandatory in all 50 states.

b. mandatory in many states.

c. at the discretion of the health care provider.

d. a matter to be handled by law enforcement agencies.

APPENDIX B

REVIEW QUESTION ANSWERS

1. Correct Answer: **D**. Radiology data alone would not be used to identify patients who may benefit from a disease management program. All other options are incorrect because they are used to identify patients who may benefit from a disease management program.

2. Correct Answer: **D**. Money is helpful but not required when the patient moves toward health and wellness. For example, spiritual wholeness does not come from having money. Option A is incorrect because knowledge is power and gives one control over one's health and wellness. Knowledge is one of the key elements needed to improve health and wellness. Option B is incorrect because to be in a position to choose better health is one of the key elements needed to improve health and wellness. This is the concept of self-determination. Option C is incorrect because empowerment to make decisions is one of the key elements needed to improve health and wellness.

3. Correct Answer: **B**. The quality department within the managed care organization is charged with reviewing any problems pertaining to network providers. Option A is incorrect because the accrediting organization that oversees the network is not structured to respond to initial complaints regarding care and has no legal authority to do so. They may discover logged complaints when reviewing documentation prior to an accreditation renewal, since this information should be part of the continuous quality review program that a managed care organization maintains. Option C is incorrect because the representative from the quality department of the managed care organization contacts the director of nursing of the home care agency to gain information during the investigation of the complaint. It is important for the case manager to follow the chain of command and to respect due process when complaints arise. Option D is incorrect because risk management does not need to be notified of a complaint unless an injury resulted from the care provided, and often the quality department is responsible for taking injury information to the risk manager. The case manager should follow the chain of command.

4. Correct Answer: **A**. Volunteer organizations are usually structured to serve large population demographics, e.g., United Way. Social service agencies are often structured for specific needs required by specific groups of people, e.g., elder services. Option B is incorrect because many social service agencies are free to eligible recipients. Option C is incorrect because both volunteer organizations and social service agencies can be funded through a variety of ways. Option D is incorrect because any volunteer organizations have paid staff members.

5. Correct Answer: **C**. The BASIS 32 is an effective health assessment screening tool for the substance abuse patient. Option A is incorrect because the ROSE health assessment screening tool is commonly used for patients with cardiac disease. Option B is incorrect because the SF36 is the most commonly used health assessment screening tool; however, it is not the best choice for the chronic alcoholic patient. Option D is incorrect because OASIS is not used as a health assessment screening tool.

6. Correct Answer: **A.** The 80/20 rule is based on a business principle that, when applied to health care, demonstrates how a small percentage of people who are affected by high-cost illnesses and injuries use a disproportionate amount of the total health care resources. Option B is incorrect because case management staffing ratios are not based on the 80/20 rule. They are usually based on the number of patients in a plan and the acuity of those patients. Option C is incorrect because a review of the literature demonstrates that the number of uninsured Americans is greater than 43 million. Option D is incorrect because the 80/20 rule does not signify the number of people covered under private insurance versus managed care. These figures continuously change.

7. Correct Answer: **B.** A situation where complications of a chronic disease are affecting activities of daily living is a crisis. The case manager must use problem-solving skills and anticipate conflict as a means to assist the noncompliant adolescent. Option A is incorrect because negotiation skills are important, but not always effective with adolescents, due to behavioral and emotional challenges inherent to this age group. Option C is incorrect because consultation with another health care professional may assist the case manager to determine an appropriate intervention, but the case manager must identify potential problems before he/she can decide whom to consult. Option D in incorrect because accountability to the patient and mother is a responsibility of the case manager. However, being accountable will not in and of itself resolve the problem.

8. Correct Answer: **A.** A hospital is a provider of services that must contain costs. The role of the acute care case manager is to ensure that patients who need to be in the hospital utilize acute care resources appropriately. Option B is incorrect because a managed care organization is not viewed as a provider, but rather as a payer. Option C is incorrect because a professional organization is a body that services a specific group of professional members. Option D is incorrect because credentialing agencies are organizations that credential providers. They usually set the standards by which providers deliver services.

9. Correct Answer: **D.** When a provider delivers a contract, he/she correctly assumes that he/she will be paid for the services rendered. Option A is incorrect because the provider has a personal choice whether to make his/her own prices competitive. Competitive pricing is not implied or guaranteed. This is generally why two or three bids should be sought by the case manager when negotiating for services. Option B is incorrect because the provider has a personal choice whether to provide quality service. There is no assurance that quality will be delivered. Option C is incorrect because the case manager should never assume that confidentiality will be maintained.

10. Correct Answer: **C.** Assessment is the first essential function in the process of case management that allows the case manager to determine a plan of care. Option A is incorrect because identification is the process used to assign a patient to case management services. Option B is incorrect because implementation involves setting a plan of care into motion after the assessment has occurred, and after the plan has been established. Option D is incorrect because coordination and interaction occur well after assignment of a new patient, and after assessment, planning and implementation.

11. Correct Answer: **D.** These are the published dietary guidelines for the patient with diabetes, according to the ADA. Option A is incorrect because these guidelines provide too little carbohydrates and too much protein for the diabetic patient. Option B is incorrect because these guidelines provide too little carbohydrates, too much protein, and too much fat for the diabetic patient. Option C is incorrect because these guidelines provide too many carbohydrates, too little protein and too little fat for the diabetic patient.

12. Correct Answer: **B.** A comprehensive rehabilitation program should be developed with an end-goal of reducing the effects a disability has on the injured or ill person's physical, emotional, and socioeconomic lifestyle. Option A is incorrect because while decreasing needed services can be a positive outcome of rehabilitation, it is not the ultimate goal of a comprehensive rehabilitation pro-

gram. Option C in incorrect because reducing costs of services is a positive outcome of rehabilitation, but should not be the ultimate goal of rehabilitation. Option D is incorrect because maximizing available services is a goal of case management. Rehabilitation should be performed in a manner that enhances the quality of life for an injured person—not to enhance a treatment plan.

13. Correct Answer: **B**. A job analysis will objectively identify the essential job functions necessary to perform the job. Option A is incorrect because a job analysis may identify potential hazards in the work area; however, its primary purpose is not to prevent further work injuries. An ergonomic evaluation would be utilized as one means to identify potential work injuries. Option C is incorrect because educational requirements necessary to perform a job are not determined in a job analysis. Educational requirements are usually identified in the job description provided by the employer. Option D is incorrect because the job market is identified in a labor market survey.

14. Correct Answer: **C**. Wrists should remain in the neutral position when typing to avoid repetitive motion injury.Option A is incorrect because flexed wrists often cause a typist to develop carpal tunnel syndrome. Option B is incorrect because extended wrists are not in the neutral position and can cause repetitive motion injury. Option D is incorrect because wrists positioned at a 45-degree angle when typing can develop carpal tunnel syndrome.

15. Correct Answer: **A**. The continuous quality improvement process in organizations depends on an efficient system to collect and analyze data, so that an objective evaluation can be made. Data are analyzed and evaluated to make changes in and to improve processes when variances occur. Option B is incorrect because data evaluated in a malpractice suit are specific to an individual case, and is not the focus of a data management system. Option C is incorrect because data evaluation as part of the billing process is completed on a case-by-case basis when denials are received from the payer of service. Option D is incorrect because the coding process is done on a case-by-case basis to ensure that all services and procedures completed in the provider setting are captured for reimbursement purposes.

16. Correct Answer: **D**. By implementing best practices, exacerbations associated with chronic illness can be decreased, but diseases are not eliminated. Option A is incorrect because by implementing best practices, case managers improve clinical outcomes. Option B is incorrect because by implementing best practices, administrative efficiencies are improved. Option C is incorrect because by implementing best practices, health care costs are reduced due to decreased fragmentation and duplication of services.

17. Correct Answer: **B**. Empowering the family toward self-care is enabling the family to meet their own needs to the greatest extent possible. Option A is incorrect because imparting medical coordination of care to family members would mean that the family is not included in the decision making process. Option C is incorrect because secondary providers may not be needed or necessary. Option D is incorrect because a grievance process must be completed by the plan member, not by the case manager. The case manager's role is to advise the plan member that he/she has a right to file a grievance and to explain the general process if necessary.

18. Correct Answer: **B**. The primary purpose of screening tools is to gain insight into patients' perceptions of their health status to identify risks early, so that treatment and compliance are maximized. Option A is incorrect because the primary use of screening tools is not to screen patients who may cost the system money, but to access patients' perceptions of their illness. Option C is incorrect because screening tools are used to evaluate patients and understand their perceptions of their health status. Option D is incorrect because screening help to identify patients who require teaching/education, but the focus of screening tools is much broader than to prevent hospitalizations.

19. Correct Answer: **D**. The patient or family or caregiver should have available contact information

in the event of equipment failure or breakdown. Option A is incorrect because instructional use of the equipment should be provided by the manufacturer's representative, usually the agency or individual delivering the equipment. Option B is incorrect because if the pay source is a third party, the case manager may not be obligated to discuss the cost of the equipment with the patient. Option C is incorrect because the ill or injured person intending to use the equipment, or a family member or caregiver, is appropriate to validate delivery of the equipment.

20. Correct Answer: **A**. The first step of resource management is to assess the patient's needs and determine achievable goals. Option B is incorrect because demand management is a process used to triage the patient to the most appropriate level of service. Option C is incorrect because evidence-based medicine is the practice of medicine that is scientifically proven to produce an expected outcome. Option D is incorrect because capitated funding pertains to one of many different methods by which health care services are paid.

21. Correct Answer: **D**. Viatical settlements are structured so that a person with six months of life expectancy may be offered 70% or more of the policy's face value, while a person with one year's life expectancy will likely be offered less. Option A is incorrect because life-care planners do not make determinations about life insurance settlements. Option B is incorrect because a living will is completed by an individual to address, while living, the issue of use or nonuse of life-sustaining procedures in the event of that person's imminent death. Whether or not a person has a living will does not legally impact the person's viatical settlement. Option C is incorrect because the viator does not negotiate with the insurance company or viatical settlement company. The amount of settlement is predetermined in accordance with a formula.

22. Correct Answer: **B**. Diagnostic testing that supports the intended procedure is needed by the UM specialist to authorize treatment. Option A is incorrect because the complete medical record is not necessary to provide pertinent medical information to authorize a plan of care. Option C is incorrect because the written order alone is not sufficient information for the UM specialist to authorize treatment. Option D is incorrect because the signed consent is necessary for the hospital to obtain, but is not supportive information that allows the UM specialist to determine that the treatment is appropriate.

23. Correct Answer: **D**. Filing an appeal through the HMO's appeal process and submitting documentation to support the medical treatment is the appropriate route for the physician to follow as a provider. Option A is incorrect because filing a lawsuit is not an option that the physician can take. A patient can file a lawsuit as the person affected by the denial. Option B is incorrect because sending a letter to the insurance commissioner is not the correct procedure. The physician would need to follow the rules for appeals established by the managed care organization. Option C is incorrect because informing the patient to file a grievance is a choice, but it will have no effect on the appeal process and would further delay the process.

24. Correct Answer: **B**. Use of utilization management and case management has been shown to result in better use of resources, cost efficiencies, and quality care. Option A is incorrect because an increase in staff credentials is not an intended outcome. Some UM and case management specialists do not have special credentials. Option C is incorrect UM and case management models do not guarantee that an overlap in administrative services will not occur. The efficiency of any organization's staff depends upon internal processes unique to the organization. Option D is incorrect because creation of a new accreditation body is not an intended outcome of UM and case management.

25. Correct Answer: **D**. The goals of a weight reduction program are to boost self-esteem, improve communication skills, improve self-confidence and promote healthy eating habits. Option A is incorrect because the goal of weight reduction programs that are designed for children do not focus on weight loss, rather they strive to boost self-esteem, improve communication skills and self-

confidence in order to achieve healthy eating habits. Option B is incorrect because weight reduction programs are geared to educate children to healthy eating habits, rather than on the negative point of view of pointing out poor eating habits. Option C is incorrect because weight reduction programs work with the individual child and their role in making healthy food choices. The parents should be involved in this process, but do not and should not control the child's diet.

26. Correct Answer: **C**. Patients who are in a disease management program are encouraged to report all positive and negative changes, since both are significant outcomes that can give important information to the team. Option A is incorrect because if a patient is adhering to the plan of care and discovers problems or changes, the patient is encouraged to call his/her treating physician to report problems. Option B is incorrect because patients involved in a disease-monitoring program are instructed to report any changes. Patients cannot typically judge which changes are significant and which are not, so that education centers on reporting any and all changes. Option D is incorrect because patients participating in disease monitoring will not be dropped from the program due to frequent admissions. Rather, the patient will receive more intense services and likely be assigned to direct case management, since frequent admissions indicate that the patient is not in control of his/her disease and needs assistance.

27. Correct Answer: **D**. Due to restrictive lung disease, patients are unable to exhale large volumes of air. Option A is incorrect because reduction of air volume and lung capacity as well as noncompliant lungs are signs of restrictive lung disease. Option B is incorrect because narrowing of airways is one of the signs of restrictive lung disease. Option C is incorrect because restrictive lung disease causes an inadequate exchange of oxygenated hemoglobin.

28. Correct Answer: **B**. A living will is intended to address end-of-life treatment issues for a person, guided by the person's own decisions when he/she is competent to make those decisions. Option A is incorrect because a living will is based on the principle of self-determination. It allows a person to legally proclaim his/her own wishes for end-of-life care in the event he/she becomes incompetent. It is not intended to protect or uphold the decisions of a person's physician. Option C is incorrect because a living will is an advance directive. Option D is incorrect because accelerated death benefits are provided by life insurance policies to make funds available to an individual prior to his/her death.

29. Correct Answer: **A**. Title III of the ADA is governed by the Department of Justice in Washington, D.C. Option B is incorrect because the Equal Employment Opportunity Commission governs Title I of the ADA. Option C is incorrect because the Architectural and Transportation Barriers Compliance Board governs Section 502 of the Rehabilitation Act. Option D is incorrect because the Department of Federal Affairs has nothing to do with the ADA.

30. Correct Answer: **C**. The portability of HIPAA allows an employee to switch jobs, even if he/she or a dependent has a chronic condition, without fear of being uninsurable or uninsured through the new employer. Option A is incorrect because former group health insurance can be maintained by a person leaving his/her employment for up to 18 months under COBRA. This would be very important if the new employer is a small business owner with no health insurance. Option B is incorrect because excluding an employee from the group plan who has a significant medical history is precisely what the HIPAA legislation prevents. Option D is incorrect because this scenario is an example of coverage available under the COBRA legislation.

31. Correct Answer: **D**. The FMLA requires employers of 50 or more employees to provide up to 12 weeks of unpaid excused leave of absence for eligible employees. Option A is incorrect because the Family and Medical Leave Act does not require employers to hold jobs open for employees for six months. Option B is incorrect because the FMLA does not require an employer to provide income to an employee during a leave of absence due to injury, illness, or birth/adoption of a baby. Therefore, it does not address taxable versus non-taxable income. Some employers do pay their

employees while on FMLA leave, but this is a decision made by the employer. Option C is incorrect because the FMLA does not require employers to provide paid leave for employees; the law mandates unpaid leave for certain circumstances.

32. Correct Answer: **A**. Subrogation allows a payer to seek recovery of benefits paid to a policy holder through the third party causing the loss. Option B is incorrect because coordination of benefits is the term used when two or more benefit plans make health care payments simultaneously. Option C is incorrect because out-of-benefit services provided to a policyholder can occur without subrogation. Out-of-benefit services means that the policy holder is covered for services not listed in the policy holder's benefit package, but made available because providing the services will save costs and enhance quality of care. Option D is incorrect because out-of-pocket expenses are those expenses incurred personally by a policy holder in accordance with his/her policy's benefit plan.

33. Correct Answer: **D**. An HMO's primary goal is to enhance the quality of care through a coordinated network. By utilizing a coordinated network, cost efficiencies can also be achieved. Option A is incorrect because the primary goal of HMOs is not to limit a patient's choice in the treatment plan. It is to enhance quality, cost-effective care. Option B is incorrect because an HMO's primary goal is not to limit benefits, but rather to effectively coordinate benefits to enhance quality care and cost savings. Option C is incorrect because an HMO's primary goal is not to limit the policyholder's section of a primary care physician. Several primary care physicians are usually available in a provider network who have a good reputation in the community, are geographically diverse, and provide various specializations.

34. Correct Answer: **B**. Correct. A person possessing an "own occ" disability policy can file a claim of wage loss under his/her policy if he/she cannot perform any aspect of his/her job. Option A is incorrect because a person possessing an "own occ" disability policy does not need to be incapable of performing all aspects of his/her job before wage loss can be implemented. Option C is incorrect because rewriting a job description and modifying the job are proactive solutions to continue working, but the "own occ" rule in disability insurance cannot dictate this opportunity. The employer is the person to determine whether he/she will re-write a job description and modify a job for an employee. Option D is incorrect because the right to sue an employer is not governed or encouraged under the "own occ" rule in disability insurance.

35. Correct Answer: **B**. Self-determination means being empowered to make one's own decisions. Confidentiality respects the right of the patient to make his/her own decisions. Option A is incorrect because self-esteem is an important aspect for the patient to achieve. However, respecting a patient's confidentiality will not boost or ensure his/her self-esteem. Option C is incorrect because self-defense is not enhanced or protected by treating the patient and his/her records confidentially. Self-defense is a person's own ability to defend himself/herself. Option D is incorrect because self-incrimination is a negative trait implying that an individual holds himself/herself accountable for an action. It is not affected by protecting confidentiality.

36. Correct Answer: **D**. A guardian is meant to oversee the person and the person's trust as established by the court. Option A is incorrect because a guardian does not mandate a person's health. Option B is incorrect because a guardian does not oversee a person's estate, although a guardian will oversee a trust established legally by the court, which would include assets that may be in the person's estate at the time of the person's death. Option C is incorrect because a guardian does not oversee "health and property". A guardian oversees "person and trusts."

37. Correct Answer: **D**. Freedom of choice by the person consenting is part of the "voluntariness" that must be present in order for an informed consent to be legal – for the patient to be informed. Option A is incorrect because although an explanation of the intended treatment is required, written documentation of the intended treatment is not required. Option B is incorrect because an explanation of what the person should expect from treatment is given verbally. This may or may

not include a timeline of when the treatment is expected to occur, as this information may not always be known at the time informed consent is being sought. Option C is incorrect because information on the outcome, verbally or in writing, cannot be given, since no one knows for sure what the outcome will be. Rather, the expected outcome should be discussed with the patient.

38. Correct Answer: **B**. Since being an informed consumer is important when purchasing health care products and services, consumers will benefit from sophisticated tools that allow them to perform comparison shopping. Option A is incorrect because consumers use sophisticated analytical tools to research information to make informed health care decisions. In the year 2030, it is expected that many consumers will pay for various health care services out of their own pockets. Networks may not even exist. Option C is incorrect because consumers in the year 2030 will use many products that improve their health and wellness that will not be found on the Internet. The Internet will be just one source for consumers. Option D is incorrect because despite sophisticated information systems and tools, a health care professional, likely the physician, will still have responsibility to diagnose and determine appropriate treatment for the patient.

39. Correct Answer: **C**. To offer value-added service to its customers to stay competitive, pharmaceuticals are offering disease management programs and on-line pharmacies. Option A is incorrect because advertising efforts are directed not just to the consumer, since health care providers also need to have this information to keep current with new treatment options. Option B is incorrect because pharmaceutical industry is using the E-health market to increase exposure of their products and services. Option D is incorrect because this is not the intent of e-health since consumers are empowered to make informed health care choices.

40. Correct Answer: **A**. Due to expected advances in technology that will occur in this century, the 21st century is termed the biotech century. Option B is incorrect because the 20th century was termed the technology century. Option C is incorrect because the year 1999 was heralded as the year of older persons, and was devoted to improving care for older persons, according to the American Society on Aging. Option D is incorrect because no century has been named as a century for reforming health care.

41. Correct Answer: **C**. Incorporating best practices makes guidelines successful. Option A is incorrect because patient requests are taken into account regarding treatment options, but are not used to develop or enact clinical guidelines. Option B is incorrect because clinical information is developed from clinical guidelines. Option D is incorrect because benchmarks result from analysis of data reported from outcomes of clinical guidelines.

42. Correct Answer: **D**. The purpose of a life-care plan is to reasonably and holistically ascertain what a catastrophically ill or injured person may require over his/her life expectancy. Option A is incorrect because life-care plans are intended to plan for a person's lifetime. A rehabilitation period may occur only during a few months of an ill or injured person's life. Option B is incorrect because life-care plans are intended to plan for a person's lifetime. The acute phase may occur only during a few weeks or months of an ill or injured person's life. Option C is incorrect because life-care plans are intended to plan for a person's lifetime. The holistic needs of a catastrophically ill or injured person do not cease 24 months after the acute phase has ended.

43. Correct Answer: **D**. Resource management can be stressful. Case managers need to focus on successes, large and small, that help patients achieve progress. Option A is incorrect because case managers do not make decisions regarding health care benefits. They can negotiate for exceptions to benefits with payers or, as the payer-based case manager, they can support existing benefit decisions. They should not see themselves as having the power to determine any individual's fate. Option B is incorrect because the patient should be the center of his/her rehabilitation process. Option C is incorrect case management is not respected by some physicians, who misunderstand

the role of the case manager to be that of policing health care dollars. Case managers depending upon respect from physicians will compound their own stress and potential burnout.

44. Correct Answer: **A**. The first step of resource management is to assess the patient's needs and determine achievable goals. Option B is incorrect because demand management is a process used to triage the patient to the most appropriate level of service. Option C is incorrect because evidence-based medicine is the practice of medicine that is scientifically proven to produce an expected outcome. Option D is incorrect because capitated funding pertains to one of many different methods by which health care services are paid.

45. Correct Answer: **C**. The Social Security Act gave federal entitlement to vocational rehabilitation as a permanent federal program in 1935. Option A is incorrect because there is not an act called the Vocational Rehabilitation and Training Act. Option B is incorrect because the SSDI program is part of the social security program and is intended to replace lost earnings from physical and mental impairments severe enough to keep an individual from working. Option D is incorrect because the Smith-Hughes Act provided funding for vocational education programs prior to enactment of permanent programs through the Social Security Act.

46. Correct Answer: **D**. The Rehabilitation Act is civil rights legislation. Option A is incorrect because the Rehabilitation Act's Section 504 requires public access in all federal buildings or by entities operating in federal locations, or funded with federal dollars. Option B is incorrect because access for all forms of public transportation is a requirement by the Americans with Disabilities Act. Option C is incorrect because the Rehabilitation Act does not govern any form of health care treatment.

47. Correct Answer: **A**. The fee-for-service insurance system focuses on paying for services and resources incurred by patients as a result of illness and injury. Preventative measures were not considered in the past fee-for-service system. Option B is incorrect because prevention was not a strategy in the past fee-for service environment. Because costs were still manageable, the need to promote wellness was not identified. Option C is incorrect because capitation is a form of economic viability established by managed care systems. Option D is incorrect because health care services in the past fee-for-service environment were not always patient oriented. Rather than promoting advocacy for patients, providers often assumed a paternalistic ("I know what's best for you") role.

48. Correct Answer: **C**. Medicare benefits are secondary benefits, with workers' compensation benefits considered the primary benefits. Option A is incorrect because Medicare benefits are secondary, while workers' compensation benefits are primary. Option B is incorrect because receiving workers' compensation benefits does not penalize a person or prevent him/her from receiving Medicare once eligible. Option D is incorrect because the Resource Based Relative Value Scale is a formula developed by Medicare to provide payments to physicians. It does not affect benefits being paid to a patient receiving workers' compensation benefits.

49. Correct Answer: **B**. Advance directives are also known as living wills. Option A is incorrect because an accelerated death benefit allows a policy holder to access his/her life insurance policy settlement prior to death. Option C is incorrect because the Patient Self-Determination Act mandates that entities inform patients of advance directives, but advance directives are not known as the Patient Self-Determination Act. Option D is incorrect because viatical settlements are a mechanism that allow the viator, or holder of a life insurance policy, to surrender his/her policy for a portion of the value of the policy. Viators are allowed to access viatical settlements when they are terminally ill.

50. Correct Answer: **B**. The reporting of abuse by anyone, whether a lay person or a health care professional or other person, is mandatory across many states in the US. Option A is incorrect because it depends upon who is reporting the abuse. Mandatory reporting by health care professionals and cer-

tain other individuals exists in all 50 states, but reporting of abuse by the lay person is only mandatory in some states. Option C is incorrect because reporting of abuse is never at the discretion of the health care provider. Option D is incorrect because law enforcement agencies and employees are required in all 50 states to report suspicion of abuse. However, many other professionals are also mandated to report abuse, such as health care professionals and school teachers.